Nutrients in the Control of Metabolic Diseases

Volume Editor

Artemis P. Simopoulos
The Center for Genetics, Nutrition and Health,
American Association for World Health, Washington, D.C.

49 figures and 26 tables, 1992

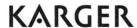

KARGER

Basel · Freiburg · Paris · London · New York · New Delhi · Bangkok · Singapore · Tokyo · Sydney

World Review of Nutrition and Dietetics

Library of Congress Cataloging-in-Publication Data
Nutrients in the control of metabolic diseases / volume editor, Artemis P. Simopoulos.
(World review of nutrition and dietetics; vol. 69)
Includes bibliographical references and index.
1. Diet in disease.   2. Non-insulin-dependent diabetes – Nutritional aspects.
3. Hypertension – Nutritional aspects.   4. Coronary heart disease – Nutritional aspects.
5. Vitamins – Pathophysiology.   6. Diet in disease – Saudia Arabia.
I. Simopoulos, Artemis P., 1933–   . II. Series.
[DNLM: 1. Metabolic Diseases – prevention & control.   2. Nutrition.]
ISBN 3–8055–5594–6

Bibliographic Indices
This publication is listed in bibliographic services, including Current Contents® and Index Medicus.

Drug Dosage
The authors and the publisher have exerted every effort to ensure that drug selection and dosage set forth in this text are in accord with current recommendations and practice at the time of publication. However, in view of ongoing research, changes in government regulations, and the constant flow of information relating to drug therapy and drug reactions, the reader is urged to check the package insert for each drug for any change in indications and dosage and for added warnings and precautions. This is particularly important when the recommended agent is a new and/or infrequently employed drug.

Nutrients in the Control of Metabolic Diseases

World Review of Nutrition and Dietetics

Vol. 69

Series Editor

Artemis P. Simopoulos, Washington, D.C.

KARGER

Basel · Freiburg · Paris · London · New York · New Delhi · Bangkok · Singapore · Tokyo · Sydney

Contents

Preface IX

Nutritional Factors and the Etiology of Non-Insulin-Dependent
Diabetes mellitus: An Epidemiological Overview
Edith J.M. Feskens, Bilthoven 1

Introduction 1
    Glucose Intolerance 2
    Heredity and Age 3
    Primary Prevention 4
Body Fatness 5
    Energy Imbalance 5
    Body Fat Distribution 13
    Etiology and Possible Prevention 15
Diet 17
    Carbohydrates and Fiber 18
    Dietary Fat and Cholesterol 20
    Dietary Protein 23
    Alcohol 24
    Micronutrients 24
Conclusion 25
Acknowledgments 26
References 26

Vitamins and Hypertension
K. Dakshinamurti, K.J. Lal, Winnipeg, Man. 40

Introduction 40
Vitamin B_6 42
    Pyridoxine Deficiency: Animal Model of Hypertension 44
    Characterization of Hypertension Induced by Vitamin B_6 Deficiency 47
Vitamin D 60

Vitamin E 65
Conclusions 66
References 67

Long-Chain ω3 Fatty Acids Are the Most Effective Polyunsaturated Fatty Acids for Dietary Prevention and Treatment of Cardiovascular Risk Factors. Conclusions from Clinical Studies

Peter Singer, Manfred Wirth, Ingrid Berger, Brigitte Heinrich, Wolfgang Gödicke, Siegfried Voigt, Berlin-Buch;
Christa Taube, Halle-Wittenberg;
Werner Jaross, Siegmund Gehrisch, Dresden

Werner Jaross, Siegmund Gehrisch, Dresden 74

Introduction 75
Slow Conversion of Linoleic and α-Linolenic Acids to Arachidonic and Eicosapen-
    taenoic Acids in Normal, Hypertensive and Hyperlipemic Subjects 75
    General Aspects 75
    Patients and Methods 77
    Results 78
    Discussion 83
Canned Mackerel as Dietary Source of Eicosapentaenoic and Docosahexaenoic
    Acids Effectively Lowers Blood Pressure, Serum Lipids, Lipoproteins and
    Thromboxane B_2 Formation in Man 84
    General Aspects 84
    Patients and Methods 86
    Results 89
    Discussion 102
Conclusion 106
References 107

The Affluent Diet and Its Consequences: Saudi Arabia – A Case in Point

Ahmed A. Al-shoshan, Riyadh

Ahmed A. Al-shoshan, Riyadh 113

Introduction 113
Overnutrition and Global Trends 114
The Middle East: A Growing Concern 119
The Kingdom of Saudi Arabia 126
    Food Production, Imports and the Availability 126
    Dietary Habits, Consumption Pattern and Available Nutrients 129
    Trends in Chronic Diseases 142

Guidelines and Recommendations 153
  The Advocacy: Administrative and Political Support 153
  The Administrative Unit: The Infrastructure 154
  Intersectoral Food and Nutrition Planning Council 154
  National Food and Nutrition Policies 156
  Development of National Dietary Guidelines 156
  Mass Media and Public Awareness 156
  Nutritional Support Unit in Primary Health Care Centers, Clinics and Hospi-
    tals 157
  Role of the Food Industry 157
  Target-Oriented Education, Training, Extension and Research Activities . . 158
  The Ultimate: You, the Individual 159
Acknowledgments 160
References 161

Subject Index 167

Preface

Advances in genetics and molecular biology have enhanced the scientific basis of nutrition. The role of nutrients in gene expression and the importance of gene-nutrient interactions in determining the health status of individuals and populations were the subjects of volume 63 of *World Review of Nutrition and Dietetics* in this series under the title *Genetic Variation and Nutrition* published in 1990. The present volume *Nutrients in the Control of Metabolic Diseases* begins with the paper on 'Nutritional Factors and the Etiology of Non-Insulin-Dependent Diabetes mellitus: An epidemiological overview'. Non-insulin-dependent diabetes mellitus (NIDDM) is a disease that involves the pathways of intermediary metabolism: in other words, a metabolic disease par excellence. Diabetes, originally described by Hippocrates, has been considered to be associated with diet since the beginning. Later on West considered obesity to be the most important nutritional factor in its etiology. Today, NIDDM is known to be a chronic disease whose onset is genetically determined depending mostly on age and obesity. This paper presents an extensive review and critique of the epidemiological evidence of body fatness in terms of energy balance and body fat distribution and the dietary factors that have been implicated in NIDDM. The studies include comparisons between populations, case-control and cross-sectional studies, cohort studies, longitudinal studies with serial measurements, intervention studies and control studies. The effects of diet include studies on carbohydrate and fiber, refined sugars (both mono- and disaccharides), polysaccharides and starch. Other dietary components reviewed are dietary fat and cholesterol, dietary protein, alcohol and micronutrients. The data suggest that, for the prevention of diabetes, energy intake, physical activity and obesity are three major components that affect glucose metabolism. Energy imbalance contributes to the development of diabetes. Specific dietary factors in the etiology of glucose intolerance point to the beneficial effects of water-soluble fiber whereas the role of simple sugars so prominent in previous studies appears to have been overestimated. Of interest is the new information about fatty acids, their role on cellular membranes and overall lipid metabolism apart from their role in the onset of abnormalities of glucose metabolism.

Hypertension is a metabolic disorder that to a great extent is also genetically determined. Lately the contributions of dietary, life-style and environmental factors to the development of hypertension has received much attention. In the second paper 'Vitamins and Hypertension', the focus is on the mechanisms of action of vitamin B_6, vitamin D and vitamin E as the only vitamins implicated in blood pressure regulation. Of these 3 vitamins, vitamin B_6 has been extensively investigated in animal models and in human beings. Pyridoxine deficiency leads to elevated blood pressure. The paper includes descriptions of studies in animals made pyridoxine-deficient in order to study the mechanisms of the development of hypertension. In these studies the role of the thyroid gland, sympathetic nervous system, central neurotransmitters, norepinephrine, serotonin and γ-aminobutyric acid are precisely described. Injection of pyridoxine reduces systolic blood pressure and sympathetic activity and also restores serotonin and γ-aminobutyric acid levels to control values. High dietary calcium prevents the hypertensive effects of vitamin-B_6-deficient diets.

Data from the US Health and Nutrition Examination Survey collected between 1971 through 1975 (NHANES I) indicate that reduced intake of calcium was the primary nutritional marker of hypertension and that the increase in systolic blood pressure correlated with a decrease in dietary calcium intake. In this paper the relationship of vitamin D metabolites, serum parathyroid hormone and serum calcium are explored in animal studies and clinical investigations. The authors conclude that epidemiological, clinical and experimental investigations all indicate a relationship between the plasma levels of $1,25\text{-}(OH)_2D_3$ and hypertension. This includes the vitamin-D-mediated significant reduction in blood pressure of hypertensives. The mechanism of the action of vitamin D in this is not understood yet. Both a direct effect, acting on cell membranes, and an indirect effect, acting through enhancement of calcium transport, are indicated.

The important role of vitamin E as a major endogenous antioxidant agent breaking the chain of lipid peroxidation in cell membranes and thus preventing the formation of lipid hydroperoxides is given particular attention in the current literature. It is also known that vitamin E stabilizes the cell membrane most likely by acting as a filler in the phospholipid bilayer. Studies show that in spontaneously hypertensive rats tissue vitamin E levels are significantly lower than in normotensive Wistar-Kyoto rat controls. Vitamin-E-deficient rats develop vascular changes similar to those found in hypertensive human preeclampsia, although blood pressure was not altered in the vitamin-E-deficient rat. Rats made deficient in vitamin E, although they do not become hypertensive, demonstrate a functional vitamin-E-deficient state by showing an increase in tissue thiobarbituric-acid-reactive material, increased pressor responsiveness to angiotension II and decreased relaxation response to acetylcholine in mesenteric arteries. These changes are seen usually in the hypertensive state.

Over the past 10 years the research on the role of ω3 fatty acids in growth and development and in health and disease has expanded throughout the world. These research advances have provided data on the essentiality of ω3 fatty acids, on the mechanisms involved in the control of risk factors for coronary heart disease by either inhibiting the development of risk factors or enhancing the development of protective factors. In the third paper on 'Long-Chain Omega-3 Fatty Acids Are the Most Effective Polyunsaturated Fatty Acids for Dietary Prevention and Treatment of Cardiovascular Risk Factors. Conclusions from Clinical Studies', a series of clinical studies are reviewed in terms of metabolic pathways involved in the elongation and desaturation of linoleic acid and linolenic acid to arachidonic acid and eicosapentaenoic acid, respectively, in normal, hypertensive and hyperlipidemic subjects. This is a most important contribution because the issue of whether α-linolenic versus eicosapentaenoic acid are effective in cardiovascular disease is dealt with here objectively. The second part of the paper deals with clinical investigations that examine precisely the effects of eicosapentaenoic acid and docosahexaenoic acid and the mechanisms involved in the control of risk factors for the prevention and treatment of cardiovascular disease.

These three papers clearly emphasize the importance of certain nutrients in the control of diabetes, hypertension and coronary heart disease. The dietary changes that have taken place in Western cultures are now also occurring in other societies. The fourth paper in this volume, 'The Affluent Diet and Its Consequences: Saudi Arabia – A Case in Point', is a most appropriate complement to this volume. It is clear that new dietary habits over a short period of time may lead to undesirable consequences unless an effort is made for the various countries and their scientific societies to consider that nutrients are important in the control of metabolic disease, and that the introduction of new nutrients may lead to maladaptation in some members of the population whose genetic constitution cannot adapt to rapid and new dietary changes. Although obesity is a most important nutritional factor in the development of NIDDM, it is the combination of increased energy intake and a sedentary life-style that need to be controlled. Similarly moderate vitamin B_6 deficiency in the presence of a decrease in calcium intake may lead to the development of hypertension in those who are predisposed to hypertension and are susceptible to it. The recent progress and research advances on the mechanisms involved in the development of cardiovascular disease make it evident that the enormous increase of vegetable oils of the ω6 fatty acid type and the decrease in ω3 fatty acid intake further contribute to hypertension. The imbalance in the ω6 to ω3 ratio resulting from the excessive intake of ω6 fatty acids and a decrease in ω3 fatty acids has shifted the physiologic state of Western populations to a state that is prothrombotic and proinflammatory which is found in patients with cardiovascular disease and diabetes, major chronic diseases of Western societies.

The papers in this volume should be of interest to physicians in all disciplines, clinical investigators, epidemiologists, dietitians, food scientists and policy makers.

Artemis P. Simopoulos, MD

Simopoulos AP (ed): Nutrients in the Control of Metabolic Diseases.
World Rev Nutr Diet. Basel, Karger, 1992, vol 69, pp 1–39

Nutritional Factors and the Etiology of Non-Insulin-Dependent Diabetes mellitus: An Epidemiological Overview

Edith J.M. Feskens

National Institute of Public Health and Environmental Protection,
Department of Epidemiology, Bilthoven, The Netherlands

Contents

Introduction   1
    Glucose Intolerance   2
    Heredity and Age   3
    Primary Prevention   4
Body Fatness   5
    Energy Imbalance   5
    Body Fat Distribution 13
    Etiology and Possible Prevention 15
Diet 17
    Carbohydrates and Fiber 18
    Dietary Fat and Cholesterol 20
    Dietary Protein 23
    Alcohol 24
    Micronutrients 24
Conclusion 25
Acknowledgments 26
References 26

Introduction

The role of diet in the etiology of glucose intolerance and non-insulin-dependent diabetes mellitus (NIDDM) is still unclear. Since long, dietary factors have been suspected to affect the development of diabetes. In 1978, West [1] concluded in his monograph that obesity was the most impor-

Table 1. Components of a chronic disease complex related to NIDDM and coronary heart disease (syndrome X), as suggested by Reaven [7]

Resistance to insulin-stimulated glucose uptake
Glucose intolerance
Hyperinsulinemia
Increased very-low-density lipoprotein triglyceride
Decreased high-density lipoprotein cholesterol
Hypertension

tant nutritional factor in the etiology of diabetes. With respect to the role of qualitative dietary factors, the epidemiological data were, however, considered to be inconclusive [1].

Glucose Intolerance

NIDDM is a chronic disease. Its onset is genetically determined, and is thought to depend mainly on age and obesity [2]. Diabetes is diagnosed from clinical symptoms or, in population studies, from results of the oral glucose tolerance test (OGTT) [2]. Nondiabetic subjects with a mild degree of glucose intolerance (impaired glucose tolerance; IGT) are found to be at higher risk for subsequent development of NIDDM [3, 4]. Recently, Saad et al. [5] postulated that the pathogenesis of NIDDM can be described by a two-step model, with IGT as an intermediate diagnosis. This glucose-intolerant state is characterized by resistance to insulin-mediated glucose uptake by the tissues and hyperinsulinemia [6–13]. Primary or secondary beta cell defects, such as islet amyloid deposition and relative beta cell exhaustion, may then lead to the development of overt diabetes. In figure 1 the possible role of insulin resistance and hyperinsulinemia in the etiology of NIDDM and glucose intolerance is summarized, as partly adapted from Zimmet [14].

Moreover, Reaven [7] recently hypothesized that insulin resistance, hyperinsulinemia and glucose intolerance form part of a chronic disease complex related to NIDDM as well as coronary heart disease, syndrome 'X' (table 1). This syndrome is recently also referred to as 'syndrome of insulin resistance' or 'metabolic syndrome', in conjunction with, e.g., central obesity [14]. Based on this syndrome, Zimmet [14] argued that NIDDM is not a discrete disease state and that, therefore, the term glucose intolerance should be preferred with respect to this risk factor complex.

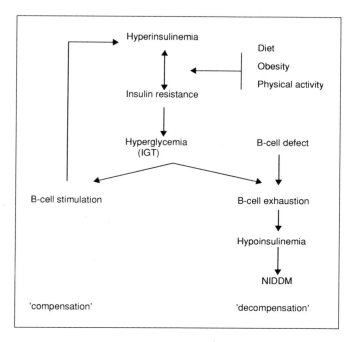

Fig. 1. Pathogenesis of NIDDM. Partly adapted from Zimmet [14]. B-cell = Beta cell.

Heredity and Age

Several aspects of the pathogenesis of diabetes depicted in figure 1 may partly be genetic in origin, such as defects of insulin sensitivity and beta cell function [9–12, 15]. Among Pacific and Asian Indian populations with generally high diabetes rates, the admixture with Caucasian genes is inversely associated with the prevalence of diabetes [16–19].

    Further epidemiological evidence for a genetic basis for glucose intolerance originates from studies on familial aggregation and twin studies mainly, although part of these results may also be explained by shared environmental factors. In several studies the prevalence and incidence of diabetes and fasting glucose levels were associated with a family history of this disease [20–24]. In studies of monozygotic twins the concordance rates for diabetes were shown to range from 55 to 100% [25, 26]. In a recent twin study the concordance rate was higher among monozygotic twins (58%) than among dizygotic twins (17%) [26]. This difference suggests that the

disease is multifactorial, and that other (environmental) factors are involved in the etiology [27]. However, the mode of inheritance is not completely clear. Also, an autosomal dominant inheritance has been suggested,
with penetrance depending on age and obesity [2]. Further investigation of
the genetics of NIDDM and glucose intolerance await the discovery of one
or more genetic markers from linkage studies in pedigrees [28]. Until now
results are, however, disappointing [29].

Age is also known as an important determinant of NIDDM. Blood
glucose levels tend to rise with age, and evidence for this aging process has
been found in many populations [1]. The deterioration of glucose tolerance
with age may be due to a decrease in both insulin sensitivity and insulin
secretion [30, 31]. This process can be inherent to aging itself. However, it
has also been suggested that the observed association with age is largely
secondary to age-related factors such as co-morbidity, medication use and
obesity [31–33].

Primary Prevention

Based on the evidence for an increased risk for the elderly and subjects
with a genetic predisposition, prevention of NIDDM may be confined to
these high-risk groups. Modifiable risk factors such as environmental and
life-style factors are, however, more important, since these are the tools for
preventive measures [14, 34].

Obesity probably is the major modifiable risk factor known to affect
the development of glucose intolerance [1, 2, 14, 24, 35]. Although obesity
may also partly be genetically determined [36, 37], it is frequently shown
that obesity and genetic susceptibility act synergistically on the development of glucose intolerance [21–24, 38]. Obesity is an indicator of energy
imbalance, reflecting the difference between energy intake and energy
expenditure [39–41]. Moreover, the distribution of fat over the body is also
a risk factor.

Diet is thought to be involved in the etiology of glucose intolerance
mainly by its association with overweight [1, 2, 35, 42]. Many experiments
have, however, shown that nutrients and foods are able to affect glucose
metabolism independently of effects on body fat [43, 44], and the first
report on this issue already dates from 1935 [45]. In addition, it is well
known that lipid metabolism and the development of cardiovascular disease are influenced by dietary factors [46, 47]. This suggests an additional
role for diet in the etiology of syndrome X and glucose intolerance, as also
indicated in figure 1. In his monograph of 1978, West [1] presented an

extensive overview of the literature, and he deduced that most epidemiological studies remained inconclusive in this respect. But several studies have been conducted since. Therefore, the more recent findings of epidemiological studies on the role of nutritional factors in the etiology of glucose intolerance will be reviewed. Overweight, body fat distribution and physical activity will be considered together with other dietary aspects. Special attention will be paid to the possible effects of preventive measures, as derived from information of prospective studies.

Body Fatness

Energy Imbalance

Time Trends. One of the oldest reports on the association between obesity and diabetes consists of observations of time trends in diabetic mortality. Already in 1875, Bourchadat noticed that diabetes rates declined during the siege of Paris, a period with food shortage [1]. Himsworth [48] reported in 1935 that diabetic mortality was reduced during World War I in countries with food rationing. Decreased mortality of diabetes was also reported during World War II, in Europe and in Japan [1]. Although in these studies no information on body weight was available, it is assumed that a large part of these observations can be ascribed to reductions in overweight [1, 42].

Comparisons between Populations. Cross-cultural studies are frequently used in epidemiological research, since they provide relatively large contrasts in exposure [49]. West and Kalbfleisch [50] showed a strong association (r = 0.89) between diabetes prevalence and mean body weight in 11 different countries. Studies of different ethnic groups within a country, such as carried out in New Zealand and the Pacific region [51–53], Israel [54] and the USA [55], showed that diabetes rates increased with increasing urbanization and modernization [51–55]. Changes in nutritional habits and physical activity accompanied these cultural processes, suggesting an association between obesity and diabetes. It must be noted that such a relationship was not observed in all populations. In some Pacific populations the association was stronger with physical activity than with overweight [52].

Several migrant studies have indicated that the cross-cultural differences could not completely be explained by hereditary factors. The prevalence of diabetes was higher in Japanese immigrants to Hawaii than in residents of Hiroshima, Japan [56, 57], higher in Indian immigrants to the UK than in India [58], and higher among migrants from Tokelau in New Zealand [59]. In the Tokelau population the increase in diabetes prevalence was accompanied by changes in body weight, energy intake, alcohol use, protein intake and physical activity [59].

Case-Control and Cross-Sectional Studies. Himsworth and Marshall [60] were some of the first investigators who carried out a case-control study on this topic, and they compared previous weight and diet between 143 diabetics and 137 controls. They noticed that diabetics had consumed diets with greater caloric content, and that 60.1% of the newly diagnosed diabetics were overweight. Comparable observations had been made by Joslin in 1921, and this was confirmed by more recent investigations on newly presenting diabetic patients in the National Health and Nutrition Examination Survey (NHANES) [61].

In the seventies, Baird [62] noticed a higher prevalence of overweight and excess energy intake in a study of 153 newly diagnosed untreated diabetic patients aged 45–65 years that were compared to their siblings and to nondiabetic siblings of control subjects. In several population studies the prevalence of diabetes, either self-reported or diagnosed by OGTT, was associated with overweight [63–69].

Since diabetics may suffer from weight loss prior to clinical diagnosis, cross-sectional studies do not always reveal an association with obesity [1]. However, several cross-sectional studies have also shown positive associations between overweight and blood glucose levels among nondiabetics. Subjects with IGT were found to have a higher body mass index (BMI) than normoglycemic subjects [70–72]. Also, within normoglycemic populations associations between BMI and fasting and postload glucose levels were observed, although correlation and regression coefficients were small [73, 74]. More recently, the association between obesity and hyperinsulinemia, well known from animal and clinical studies [6, 75], has also been shown in population-based studies [76–81].

Few studies have investigated physical activity or energy intake in this respect. Chen and Lowenstein [66] observed an inverse association between physical activity and the prevalence of diabetes especially in older participants of the NHANES I, but this may reflect therapeutic behavior. In the Tecumseh Study no association between habitual physical activity and glucose tolerance was observed in the total study population, except for the leanest men [82]. Among young adults from the Beaver County Study, insulin sensitivity and physical activity were positively, but not significantly, associated [78].

It must be noted that in addition to physical activity also physical fitness may be important in chronic disease etiology. Several studies showed that fitness was an independent risk factor for ischemic heart disease [83, 84], and physical fitness, as assessed by maximal oxygen uptake, was inversely associated with postload insulin during an OGTT in a small population of 133 men [85].

Physical activity has also been shown to be partly reflected by energy intake relative to body weight [86, 87]. Indeed, this may be an explanation for the frequently observed inverse association between energy intake and BMI [41, 88]. Energy intake was inversely associated with glucose levels in two British large-scale studies, but this could largely be accounted for by a relationship with overweight [89]. In a study of male employees, energy intake was, however, inversely associated with fasting and postload insulin levels, independently of BMI [90]. Thus, it is clear that the close relationship between the different aspects of energy imbalance hampers the interpretation of the observed results: the separate effects are difficult to disentangle.

Cohort Studies. From prospective studies the risk of the development of NIDDM and glucose intolerance with increased obesity can be assessed. Since the early seventies several studies have been reported, although many studies were not specifically designed to investigate the association between obesity and incidence of diabetes. The results of these cohort studies are summarized in table 2. In our overview one retrospective cohort was included [100]. Almost all studies showed an increased risk of diabetes with increasing BMI or relative body weight, also independently of major confounders such as age. The largest study showed a striking continuous risk gradient of diabetes risk with BMI overweight, with the lowest risk observed for a BMI below 22 kg/m^2 [24].

The various results are not easy to compare. Different methods and criteria were used to define overweight and the population at risk and to diagnose diabetes. The origin of the populations differed, and the general incidence rate varied from 0.4/1,000 person-years in US alumni [92] to 27.1/1,000 person-years in Pima Indians [21]. However, the summary of the results presented in table 2 indicates that the relative risk for NIDDM associated with overweight ranged from 1.5 to 58, with the highest risks

Table 2. Summary of results of cohort studies on overweight and incidence on diabetes mellitus (NIDDM)

Study, reference	Study period	Follow-up years	Sex	Age years	Total number
Norway, 91		10	M	40–49	3,670
US, 92	1916–1966	16–50	M	student	26,446
Israelic Ischemic Heart Disease Study, 93	1963–1968	5.0	M	20+	9,462
Pima Indians, US, 21	1965–	6.0	M/F	5–94	3,137
Paris Protective Study, France, 94	1967–1972	4.4	M	43–54	7,362
Tecumseh Study, US, 95	1959–1979	16.0	M/F	20–55+	3,881
Nauru, Polynesia, 96	1975–1982	6.5	M/F	< 19–60+	266
Gothenburg, Sweden, 97	1967–1980	13.5	M	54	766
Framingham Heart Study, US, 98	1971–1982	8.0	M/F	40–79	2,281
Israel Study of Glucose Intolerance, Obesity and Hypertension, 99	1969–1982	10	M/F	28–57	2,140
The Netherlands, 100	1967–1983	11	M/F	20–50	1,953
Gothenburg, Sweden, 101	1968–1981	12.0	F	38–60	1,462
Zutphen Study, The Netherlands, 102	1960–1985	25.0	M	40–59	841
Rancho Bernardo, US, 103	1972–1987	12.0	M/F	40–79	1,847
San Antonio Heart Study, US, 104	1979–1987	8.0	M/F	25–64	474
Nurses' Health Study, US, 24	1976–1984	8.0	F	30–55	113,861

BMI is given in kilograms per square meter. AP_c = Attributable proportion, calculated retrospectively from data at hand; RW = relative weight; RR = relative risk; RD = risk difference; diff. = difference in baseline BMI between incident cases and non-cases;

Cases	Incidence n/1,000 p-y	Diabetes diagnosis	Obesity diagnosis	Effect	APc
44	1.2	clinical	RW > 10%	RR 5.3 RD 2.2/1,000	0.57
395	0.4	clinical	BMI < 23.2 > BMI	RR 1.5 diff. 0.5	0.11
373	8.0	GTT	BMI < 24–27 > BMI	RR 2.5 RD 7.2/1,000 diff. 1.3	0.33
340	27.1	GTTs	BMI 25–30/20–25 BMI 30–35/20–25	RR 1.6 RD 6.4/1,000 RR 7.4	0.31 0.64
174	5.4	GTTs	BMI < 24.5–27 > BMI	RR 6.2 RD 8.8/1,000 diff. 2.9	
190	3.1	GTT	RW M F	diff. 14.3 diff. 21.3	
27	16.4	GTTs	BMI M F	diff. 3 diff. 6	
47	4.7	GTTs	BMI < tertile > BMI	RR 6.4 diff. 2.6	0.57
93	5.2	GTT	BMI M F	diff. 1.8 diff. 4.0	
132	6.4	GTTs	BMI < 27 >	RR 2.4 RD 7.1/1,000	0.24
35	1.6 5.6	clinical	BMI < 26 > M F	5.2	
43	2.5	clinical	BMI	diff. 5.8	
58	4.8	clinical	BMI < 22–26 > BMI	RR 2.4 RD 2.2/1,000 diff. 1.0	0.26
219	10.5	GTTs	BMI < quartile > M F	RR 1.5 RR 3.0	0.11 0.33
28	7.6	GTTs	BMI < 27 > BMI	RR 2.0 RD 4.9/1,000 diff. 3.2	0.20
873	0.9	clinical	BMI < 27 > < 3–97% >	RR 8.0 RR 58	0.58

GTT = clinical/screening glucose tolerance test; GTTs = GTT comparable to recent standards and criteria.

observed for the most overweight subjects. An overall risk ratio can be estimated from the studies by weighing according to the variances of the effect estimates [105]. For moderate overweight (BMI 25–30 kg/m^2) this results in a value of 2.6. Because of the different methodologies used, this result must be interpreted as a general estimate and regarded carefully. For more obese subjects higher relative risks were reported [24, 97].

The absolute difference in risk between categories of body weight gives an impression of the size of the public health problem in the various populations [106]. As recalculated from the data at hand, this difference varied from 1/1,000 to 10/1,000 person-years, with an intermediate value of 5/1,000 person-years. In addition, the proportion of all diabetes cases in the populations that can be attributed to overweight can be derived from the attributable proportion. The attributable proportion is calculated from information on the relative risk and the prevalence of obesity [106]. From table 2 it can be derived that this varies from 11% for elderly US men to 64% for Pima Indians, with an intermediate value of about 30%. If causality of the relation between overweight and diabetes is assumed, it can be inferred that for middle-aged Caucasian populations about 30% of the NIDDM incidence can be prevented by reducing the BMI below 25 kg/m^2. Again, this estimate must be interpreted carefully, as it strongly depends on the causal model of the disease etiology and, therefore, on the prevalence of other etiologic factors of the disease [107]. It must also be noted that several studies investigated men and women separately, showing that the effect of overweight is somewhat higher in women than in men (table 2). Only in one study was the effect of BMI adjusted for energy intake or physical fitness as reflected by resting heart rate, but this did not affect the effect estimate [102]. Whenever investigated, the results for overweight were also independent of a positive family history [21, 24].

Most of the reported prospective studies focused on diabetes mellitus (NIDDM). In a small Dutch elderly cohort it was shown that the BMI was also related to the incidence of IGT, with relative risks comparable to those reported in former studies [108]. In studies of Swedish middle-aged men [97], Israeli adults [99] and US elderly [103] the incidence of IGT was also related to baseline BMI, but the observed relative risks were smaller than observed for the incidence of diabetes.

Among subjects with IGT the effect of overweight is less clear. BMI was related to worsening of diabetes only after 5 years of follow-up in the Bedford Survey [109]. In the Whitehall Study the IGT subjects with future diabetes had a higher BMI (+1 kg/m^2), but this difference was not statistically significant in this relatively small sample (n = 181) [3]. Among Pima Indians with IGT, a BMI $> 27 \, kg/m^2$ was associated with a 2.9 times higher risk for development of NIDDM [110]. Among a Japanese population of IGT subjects the mean BMI was associated with the development of diabetes, but not independently of baseline glucose and insulin [4]. It must, however, be noted that the full effect of overweight may not be shown after adjustment for possible intermediates [106], such as glucose levels.

Besides the amount of overweight, also the duration and maximal overweight have been suggested to be associated with an increased risk of diabetes [111]. Among Pima Indians the duration of obesity was related to the risk of diabetes independently of concurrent obesity [112]. The same study showed also that former weight gain was not an independent predictor when current BMI was taken into account. However conditional upon initial BMI at age 18, weight gain was a strong risk factor for the risk of diabetes in a large study of US nurses [24]. Apparently, adult weight gain is important, at least as far as it results in higher body weight later in life.

The effect of physical activity and energy intake was only addressed in a few studies. Feskens and Kromhout [102] showed that energy intake or energy intake per kilogram body weight was not clearly related to diabetes incidence in middle-aged men, but an association with resting heart rate was noticed independently of, e.g., BMI. Resting heart rate was also a prognostic factor for the 5-year incidence of diabetes in Israeli men [113]. Since heart rate is inversely associated with physical activity and fitness [46, 114], these results suggest an additional effect of physical activity on diabetes risk. Finally, in two recent prospective studies physical activity was inversely associated with the incidence of self-reported diabetes [115, 116]. In the 14-year follow-up of surviving alumni the effect of physical activity could only partly be explained by body weight change [116].

In the prospective studies summarized in table 2, also other determinants for diabetes were investigated. Skinfold thickness [95, 102], serum total cholesterol [93, 96, 103], high-density and very-low-density lipoprotein cholesterol [98], serum triglycerides [94, 96, 103], systolic blood pressure [92–94, 98, 102, 103], liver dysfunction [94], smoking [96, 102], diuretic use [98], peripheral vascular disease [93, 98], vital capacity [92] 'and uric acid level [93, 96, 97] were all factors associated with the incidence of diabetes. Some of these associations, such as with systolic blood pressure, serum cholesterol and serum triglycerides, could largely be explained by associations with overweight.

Longitudinal Studies with Serial Measurements. The change in glucose levels associated with changes in body weight has been investigated in several longitudinal studies. Analyses of data from the Framingham Heart Study [117] showed that weight gain was associated with blood glucose elevations, although the regression coefficients were not statistically significant for all subpopulations, especially among the elderly. The proportion of variance explained by changes in relative weight was below 3%. Among Swedish middle-aged women, weight gain was associated with an increase in fasting glucose levels, also with low explained variance (0.8%): the results indicated that fasting levels increased with 0.016 mmol/l for every kilogram body weight gain [118]. In the Normative Aging Study [119], 1% of weight gain was associated with an increase of 0.051 mmol/l in 2-hour glucose and of 0.019 mmol/l in fasting glucose, with 1% of the variance explained. However, some effect modification by age was noticed in this study: among the elderly participants the effect of weight gain on fasting glucose levels was stronger than among participants of middle age. Among elderly men and women in the Netherlands [120], 1 kg body weight gain was associated with an increase of 7 mmol/l·min in the area under the curve, comparable to 0.055 mmol/l in 2-hour glucose.

Apparently, a longitudinal (age-related) increase in fasting and post-load glucose levels can only to a minor extent be explained by an increase in body weight, and the effect estimates are small. Despite, however, the differences in age and sex, the results of the various studies show a remarkable consistency and are strongly statistically significant.

Intervention Studies and Controlled Trials. Intervention trials may give further evidence that glucose levels and the risk of diabetes can indeed be reduced by a weight loss. Subjects with IGT are known to be at a higher risk for developing diabetes, and they are, therefore, likely candidates to be studied in this respect [121]. To date, however, only few trials addressed the prevention of diabetes in IGT. Since the effect of diet or weight loss and medication use was investigated simultaneously in these studies, no separate conclusion on weight loss or diet can be drawn. No effects of diet and/or treatment with oral hypoglycemic agents were observed in two small British studies [3, 89], whereas in a Swedish study a significant smaller diabetes rate was observed in IGT subjects treated with diet and/or medication [122].

In addition, it must be noted that the two-step pathogenesis model of NIDDM implies that the factors involved in the development of NIDDM from IGT merely affect the beta cell exhaustion (fig. 1). Studies of the prevention or postponement of insulin resistance should, therefore, also involve normoglycemic subjects. Again, only few of such intervention studies have been carried out. One study consisted of a cardiovascular prevention program, with 150 middle-aged men who received dietary recommendations to reduce serum cholesterol levels and overweight [123]. In this study, weight loss by a diet low in cholesterol and saturated fat resulted in a significant decrease in fasting and postload glucose levels, compared to participants not losing weight. In a smaller experimental study, weight loss achieved by dietary measures improved glucose tolerance in 20 obese men aged 46–73 years, whereas the effect of a physical training program was less strong, possibly since body fatness was not affected [124]. In normoglycemic men, exercise is thought to affect mainly the insulin resistance, and benefits on glucose tolerance may then only be observed in the long term [125, 126].

Further evidence of beneficial effects on glucose metabolism of changes in weight or physical activity originates from interventions among diabetic patients. In general, beneficial effects of reduced energy intake or increased exercise are shown [127–129]. Reduced caloric intake and regular exercise are, therefore, recommended for obese diabetic patients [130].

Although controlled trials are suitable to evaluate the effects of intervention and preventive measures, the few number of studies conducted indicate that serious difficulties are encountered using this study design. Similar to many trials concerning other diseases [49], the main problems in this respect consist of the large sample size required, the dietary compliance, the long duration of the study required and the ethical aspects. Therefore, probably only a few additional studies can be expected to be conducted in the future.

Body Fat Distribution

Besides general obesity, the regional distribution of fat over the body may induce an additional risk for the development of NIDDM. Vague [131] was the first to report that in diabetics a male type of subcutaneous fat pattern, called android or upper-body obesity, was found more often than a female type of fat pattern (gynoid or lower obesity). As an index of fat distribution he used the index of masculine differentiation, composed of the nape/sacrum skin fold ratio, and the brancho/femoral adipo-musculo ratio, derived from skin fold and circumference measurements of arm and thigh.

Other measurements of skin fold thickness have been used to discern fat patterning over the body, and they were confirmed to be strongly associated with glucose intolerance. Compared to nondiabetics, diabetics had more subcutaneous fat on the trunk [132–134]. Subcutaneous trunk fat, and notably subscapular skin fold thickness, was also associated with fasting and postload blood glucose and insulin levels in young and old populations [72, 74, 134–136]. Finally, in three prospective studies the subscapular skin fold thickness was the indicator for body fatness that was most strongly associated with diabetes incidence compared to BMI and other skin fold thicknesses [95, 102, 104].

In more recent studies, also the ratio of waist to hip or thigh circumference (WHR) was used to discern upper- and lower-body obesity. One advantage is its greater precision when standardized methods are employed [137]. In addition, the WHR primarily takes the intra-abdominal fat depot into account [138, 139]. This fat depot has especially been shown to play an important role in the metabolic disorders related to obesity [140]. In several studies it was found that the WHR was related to fasting and postprandial glucose and insulin levels, hemoglobin A_{1c}, and to the prevalence as well as the incidence of NIDDM [69, 104, 115, 141–150].

It must be noted that among female Mexican Americans the WHR as well as the subscapular to triceps skin fold ratio were associated with the prevalence of NIDDM in women independently of each other [151]. In two studies on body circumferences in women it was shown that breast circumference was also related to diabetes prevalence and serum insulin independently of overweight [80, 146]. In addition to the results from other studies concerning subscapular skin folds, this suggests that different aspects of fat patterning, central and abdominal obesity, can be discerned, having different or additional metabolic consequences.

The metabolically most detrimental fat depot, also regarding glucose metabolism, is probably the visceral fat depot that consists mostly of omental and mesenteric fat. In the study of Després et al. [152] glucose tolerance, but not the insulin or C peptide level, was independently associated with deep abdominal fat as assessed with computed tomography (CT scan) in 52 women. In this study, insulin and C peptide levels were more strongly associated with trunk skin fold thickness. In a study of 146 Japanese Americans the intra-abdominal fat area from a CT scan was a main predictor of diabetes incidence [153]. All studies regarding these intra-abdominal fat depots included only a limited number of participants, since nuclear magnetic resonance or CT scans are costly to produce.

Although the WHR does not discern between visceral and subcutaneous abdominal fat, it remains the most practical tool to assess abdominal body fat distribution in epidemiological studies. In addition, skin fold and other circumference measurements supply information on central- or upper-body obesity. The sagittal diameter has recently been proposed as a superior indicator of the visceral fat depot [154], but this remains to be confirmed in future studies.

Etiology and Possible Prevention

There still remain some controversies regarding the direction of the associations among the triad obesity, insulin resistance and hyperinsulinemia, as depicted in figure 1. It has been suggested that hyperinsulinemia may be primary as well as secondary to insulin resistance [6–13]. Some authors have also suggested hyperinsulinemia to be a cause rather than a result of obesity [14]. The metabolic and epidemiological studies investigating the detrimental effects of body fat distribution have shed more light on the underlying pathology. The relations seem to be complex, and it may well be that different diabetic disease entities exist [5, 14].

According to Kissebah and Peiris [155], overall obesity moderately reduces peripheral and hepatic insulin sensitivity, with a moderate increase in insulin secretion as secondary phenomenon to overcome this resistance. Upper (or central)-body fat obesity results in more pronounced resistance to insulin in the various tissues, and thereafter the peripheral insulin response to maximal insulin concentrations and the hepatic insulin extraction are reduced. In obese subjects a defect of the cellular insulin receptor has indeed been frequently shown [156]. Also postreceptor defects have been noticed, resulting in a variety of cellular abnormalities [156]. Part of these may well be genetically determined [141].

There is also evidence that the origin of insulin resistance is metabolic in nature. Already in the sixties it was suggested that an increased supply of free fatty acids (FFA) to peripheral (muscle) tissues can restrain glucose transport and intracellular glucose disposal [157]. Due to this substrate competition, insulin action on glucose could be impaired, secondary to a derangement in lipid metabolism. The close connnection with peripheral insulin resistance may thus be the reason for subcutaneous central-body fat to be strongly related to glucose metabolism and diabetes risk.

Others have also acknowledged an important role for FFA, albeit primarily by inducing hyperinsulinemia in relation to intra-abdominal fat [140]. These fat depots have been shown to be highly lipolytic, and to be relatively insensitive to antilipolytic action of insulin. The higher FFA concentrations in the portal vein in persons with central obesity results in a higher hepatic exposure of FFA. Besides an increase in the hepatic secretion of very-low-density lipoprotein, this may result in an increased gluconeogenesis, a reduction of hepatic insulin clearance and possibly also inhibition of insulin-stimulated glucose uptake by the tissues. The resulting hyperinsulinemia could induce insulin resistance by so-called down-regulation of the receptors. Peiris et al. [158] reported that general obesity was associated with increased insulin secretion, whereas abdominal obesity was specifically associated with a reduced clearance of insulin.

According to others, hyperinsulinemia, and not obesity-linked insulin resistance, is the main cause of derangements in carbohydrate (and lipid) metabolism as well as obesity [14]. In the sixties, Neel [159] already proposed the so-called 'thrifty-genotype' hypothesis to explain the increased obesity and diabetes in populations with increasing 'westernization' of life-style. During famine, survival is improved by hyperinsulinemia, hypertriglyceridemia and glucose intolerance. But with increasing affluence these characteristics become deleterious [160]. This may explain the high prevalence rates of obesity and diabetes in some Indian and Polynesian populations.

Although different hypotheses have been suggested, it is clear that insulin resistance and hyperinsulinemia need to be prevented to reduce glucose intolerance risk. However, the etiology of general obesity is far from elucidated. Genetic susceptibility, hormonal and neurological factors, energy overnutrition and reduced energy expenditure have all been associated with the onset of overweight, which is likely to be multifactorial in origin [40]. Hypocaloric diets such as very-low-calorie diets have been increasingly used in the treatment of obesity, and they were shown to improve glycemic control in diabetic patients [127, 129, 161]. Theoretically, also a reduced fat intake should prevent the onset of obesity [39, 40], but epidemiological and experimental evidence for this is limited. In one population-based study, fat intake was shown to be associated with body fat percentage [162]. These results, however, need further confirmation.

For the prevention of NIDDM and glucose intolerance the modifiable determinants of body fat distribution are of additional interest. Several factors have been thought to increase fat accumulation in the abdomen apart from genetic background. Especially increased androgenicity and levels of glucocorticosteroids were shown to be associated with abdominal fatness [140]. Potentially preventable life-style factors such as smoking, alcohol use and stress are hypothesized to affect fat distribution also by mediating glucocorticosteroids. In fact, Björntorp [140] suggested hypothalamic arousal to be the primary factor responsible for insulin resistance and its related metabolic syndrome (table 1), interacting with obesity. This has been suggested before [163, 164].

Evidence from epidemiologial studies for these hypotheses is yet scarce. Regarding smoking three studies showed a positive association with WHR, independently of BMI [165–167]. Furthermore, smoking was an independent risk factor for incidence of diabetes among middle-aged men, independently of potential confounders such as BMI, subscapular skin fold thickness and resting heart rate [102]. In contrast, smoking was inversely associated with 1-hour insulin levels in a cross-sectional study [168]. It is also well established that smoking is associated with reduced body weight, due to elevated resting metabolism [169]. Thus, although smoking is known to affect the sympathetic nervous system [170], and therefore metabolism, the effects on obesity and glucose metabolism are still unclear. A role of the sympathetic nervous system may also partly explain the observed association between resting heart rate and diabetes risk [102, 113]. This remains, however, to be confirmed by future studies.

The effects of alcohol on body fat distribution are still unclear [167], although in one cohort of this international study an association between γ-glutamyltransferase levels and body fat distribution was observed [171]. It must be noted that also the epidemiological association between alcohol use and obesity was recently reviewed and found to be conflicting [172].

Whether increased physical activity or dietary changes are able to affect the fat distribution over the body apart from general overweight also remains to be elucidated. Among Mexican Americans the WHR was not clearly associated with any behavioral variable [173]. However, in a small intervention study it was shown that weight reduction by dietary restriction reduced the WHR in obese women [174]. In addition, an inverse association between physical activity and WHR was observed in a study of European men [167]. Further information on this issue is awaited from future studies.

Diet

Numerous experimental studies have shown short- as well as long-term effects of specific nutrients on glucose metabolism in normal and diabetic subjects. In fact, the recent dietary recommendations for diabetic patients are mainly based on these results [130]. However, results from epidemiological studies were considered inconclusive [1, 42]. This may be partly due to methodological problems, such as the quality of the dietary assessment, or the lack of power to detect a presumably small relative risk [49]. It must also be noted that in cross-sectional surveys the association between habitual food intake and diabetic status is confounded by the use of prescribed diets. An important additional problem in nutritional epidemiology is the distribution of the dietary intake within a population. In general, within populations the range of 'exposure' is quite small. Therefore, associations with disease outcomes, such as diabetes or coronary heart disease, may not be observed [46].

Recently, some progress has been made in this area by using more reliable methodology to obtain dietary information, and by studying elderly populations with a relatively high prevalence and incidence of glucose intolerance. In addition, information was obtained on glucose tolerance rather than on clinically diagnosed diabetes. As shown in figure 1, diet is probably primarily involved in the onset of insulin resistance rather than beta cell failure, and may therefore be more closely related to IGT than to NIDDM.

Carbohydrates and Fiber

Carbohydrates are known to be strong potentiators of beta cell activity, and have therefore been suspected to influence glucose tolerance and diabetes since many years. Himsworth [45] suggested in 1935 that insulin sensitivity increased on a high-carbohydrate diet, and this is still the basis of a standard recommendation regarding the dietary preparation for the OGTT procedure. He also compared data on national diabetic mortality and dietary studies of various countries, showing an inverse association with the energy density of carbohydrates [48]. In addition, he noticed that in periods of food rationing and increased relative contribution of carbohydrates to the diet the national diabetic mortality rates decreased [48]. In the international survey of West and Kalbfleisch [50] an inverse association between carbohydrate consumption and the prevalence of diabetes was shown. With respect to within-population studies, an inverse association between carbohydrate intake and glucose levels was recently observed in US men [134]. In a British study of 220 adults, carbohydrate intake was inversely associated with fasting insulin and the area under the insulin curve, but this association was not independent of energy intake [90]. In contrast, in a study of elderly men and women the energy density of total carbohydrates was positively associated with the 4-year risk of glucose intolerance [108]. Thus, until now the effect of total carbohydrates is unclear.

However, more recent experimental studies have shown that the intake of different carbohydrate foods results in different glycemic responses [43, 44, 175–184]. Especially the simple sugars have been thought to affect diabetes detrimentally [181, 185, 186]. In contrast, the intake of starch and polysaccharides was suggested to have beneficial effects, partly due to their association with fiber intake [187]. It is, therefore, important to consider the different types of carbohydrates separately.

Refined Sugars/Mono- and Disaccharides. In his monograph of 1978, West [1] described the controversy concerning sugars from studies up to that time. Since the past century, 21 studies had suggested that sugars were involved in the etiology of diabetes, whereas 22 studies were cited not to have observed this. In two additional cross-sectional studies, sugar intake was shown to be inversely associated with fasting and postload glucose levels [89, 188]. Obese subjects are known to underestimate their sugar intake [189], but after adjustments for BMI and energy intake the results remained essentially the same [188]. In a prospective study of Israeli men the intake of sucrose was also inversely related to the subsequent diabetes incidence, but this result was not independent of energy intake and body fatness [190]. In contrast to these inverse relationships, in a recent prospective study among an elderly population the use of pastries identified a group of subjects being at a higher risk of developing glucose intolerance [108]. In this study no overall association with mono- and disaccharides or sugar was noticed.

In experimental studies an acute blood glucose reduction was shown after sugar intake [44]. This is at least partly caused by an increased insulin secretion, which can eventually give rise to hyperinsulinemia [181], and thus possibly to NIDDM (fig. 1). It must, however, be noted that in several long-term experiments on healthy subjects no unfavorable effects of physiologic amounts of sucrose on glucose metabolism were observed [175, 176, 191]. Thus, concerning the consumption of sugar as a risk factor, a definite conclusion can apparently not yet be drawn. Future studies, including insulin measurements, may clarify these paradoxical results.

Starch, Polysaccharides and Fiber. The glycemic response of starchy foods has been shown to depend on the fiber content, and especially on the content of water-soluble fiber [44, 192]. The glycemic index is an index of acute glycemic response. In general, the glycemic index of carbohydrate foods containing water-soluble fiber is low [44]. Although most studies addressed the short-term glucose response to foods, also the long-term use of soluble fiber foods has been shown to result in lower glucose levels during OGTT [184, 193, 194]. The beneficial effect of water-soluble dietary fibers, like pectin and guar, were observed among healthy as well as among diabetic individuals [177, 179, 180, 182]. The effect of wheat fiber was less strong [179].

Several mechanisms for the beneficial effect of soluble fibers on glucose metabolism have been suggested, such as the delay of gastric emptying [177, 182, 194]. Also an increased insulin sensitivity of the tissues was reported, possibly due to effects on gastrointestinal hormone secretion [180].

Epidemiological evidence for a beneficial effect of fiber consisted mainly of an ecologic study by Trowell [187]. This study concerned total fiber only. Additional evidence was, however, published recently. In a cross-sectional study of normoglycemic middle-aged men the intake of pectin was inversely associated with postload glucose levels, independently of potential confounders such as energy intake and BMI [188]. Also the consumption of legumes, characterized by a high content of water-soluble fiber, was inversely associated with the risk of glucose intolerance [108]. This was the first prospective study confirming the beneficial effects of the aforementioned experimental and cross-sectional studies.

It is conceivable that effects of polysaccharides merely originate from their association with dietary fibers. It must, however, be noted that among Pima Indians the use of polysaccharides was positively associated with the incidence of NIDDM [195]. But the interpretation of these results is hampered by the lack of adjustment for BMI.

Dietary Fat and Cholesterol

Several decades ago, Himsworth [48] observed that higher diabetes rates occurred in populations with a relatively high fat intake (fig.2). More recently, West and Kalbfleisch [50] noticed a positive association between fat consumption and diabetes rates in an international survey. It can be argued that these associations are due to positive associations with total energy intake or sucrose, or to inverse associations with carbohydrates. However, results of several experiments suggest that, besides carbohydrates and fiber, also fat intake may affect tissue insulin sensitivity and hepatic glucose output, even apart from effects on body fatness [183, 196, 197].

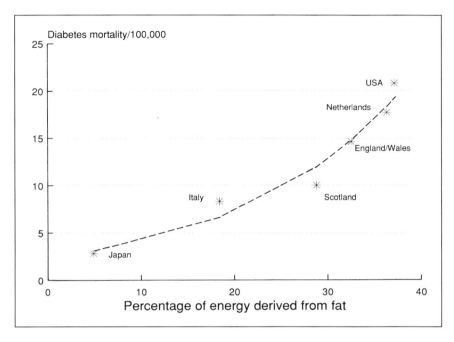

Fig. 2. National diabetes mortality rates by percentage of energy derived from fat, 1935 [45].

Further epidemiological evidence that the total fat intake is related to carbohydrate metabolism is scarce. The source of fat may, however, be more important, comparable to known effects on lipid metabolism. In a population of Seventh-Day Adventists, meat consumption was observed to be an independent risk factor for diabetes mortality [198]. This suggests a detrimental effect of saturated fatty acids. Saturated fatty acids and dietary cholesterol were also positively related to fasting and postprandial glucose levels in normoglycemic men, independently of energy intake and body fatness [188]. In a recent Italian population study, butter consumption was positively associated with fasting glucose levels, whereas an inverse association with the use of olive oil was observed [199]. In study on healthy young men it was observed that the polyunsaturated to saturated fatty acid ratio in phospholipids was inversely associated with insulin secretion and positively related to insulin action [200]. Finally, in a small sample of Japanese Americans with IGT it was shown that the intake of animal fat, probably by its association with intake of saturated fatty acids, was related to the progression to NIDDM [201]. A preceding cross-sectional analysis of the diet of normal and diabetic Japanese Americans had also revealed a positive association with animal fat intake [202].

ω3 polyunsaturated fatty acids have also been suggested to be involved in disorders of glucose metabolism [203]. This hypothesis initially originated from the observed low incidence of diabetes in populations consuming large amounts of fish and marine foods, e.g. Greenland and Alaskan Eskimos and Alaskan Indians [204, 205]. Apparently, these findings could not be explained by differences in genetic predisposition or obesity. More importantly, in a recent prospective study among 175 elderly men and women it was shown that habitual fish eaters had about a 50% lower risk to develop glucose intolerance over a subsequent 4-year period [206].

Results of in vitro studies support the suggestion that fatty acids play a role in glucose metabolism. Compared to ω6 polyunsaturated fatty acids, saturated fatty acids have been shown to decrease cellular insulin response in several experiments [207, 208]. ω3 polyunsaturated fatty acids are known to alter the production of eicosanoids, which may modulate beta cell activity [209].

Additional evidence for a relation between dietary fatty acids and carbohydrate metabolism can be derived from intervention studies among diabetic patients. In a controlled intervention study, the isocaloric replacement of linoleic acid by saturated fatty acids resulted in an increase in blood glucose levels and insulin requirements [210]. In obese diabetic patients replacement of carbohydrates and saturated fatty acids by ω6 polyunsaturated fatty acids resulted in lower glucose and insulin levels [211]. Beneficial effects were also shown in a study of longer duration [212]. However, in a study of 14 NIDDM patients the increase of the polyunsaturated to saturated fatty acid ratio of the diet from 0.3 to 1.0 did not result in a clear effect on glucose metabolism, although an increase in the in vitro insulin binding and metabolic clearance rate of glucose was reported [213]. In this respect it must be noted that a recent experimental study with rats showed that the effect of dietary changes in fatty acids is relative to the basic fat content of the diet [214]. This important issue requires further investigation.

Beneficial effects of other fatty acids have also been shown in an experimental setting. In a study of 10 NIDDM patients the partial replacement of complex carbohydrates by monounsaturated fatty acids resulted in lower mean plasma glucose levels and reduced insulin requirements [215]. Storlien et al. [216] observed an increased insulin sensitivity in liver tissue and skeletal muscle when dietary ω6 polyunsaturated fatty acids were partially replaced by fish oil in rats. In rats on a fish oil diet a lower incidence of diabetes was noticed compared with a control group [217]. Addition of 6 g ω3 polyunsaturated fatty acids to the diet of 8 normal volunteers resulted in significant increase in insulin sensitivity [218].

Thus, the effects of dietary fatty acids on glucose tolerance now observed in experimental as well as epidemiological studies are largely comparable to known effects of fatty acids on serum lipids [46, 47, 219]: detrimental effects of saturated fatty acids were shown, whereas beneficial effects of mono- and polyunsaturated fatty acids were reported. This suggests a common etiology, in agreement with the recent hypothesized metabolic syndrome (syndrome X; table 1).

The beneficial effect of ω3 polyunsaturated fatty acids can be partly due to their known potential to decrease very-low-density lipoprotein triglyceride synthesis [214, 220]. This may affect the balance in cellular fuel uptake, possibly resulting in enhanced glucose clearance by the so-called Randle cycle [157]. Furthermore, the incorporation of polyunsaturated fatty acids in cellular membranes affects the fluidity of the membranes. This stimulates the activity of insulin receptors and glucose transport, and increases insulin sensitivity of the tissues [214, 221]. In a study of 356 children it was shown that the fluidity of the erythrocyte membrane was associated with high-density to low-density lipoprotein cholesterol levels as well as with postload glucose levels [222]. This implies that the association between lipid and carbohydrate metabolism is also partly mediated by the fluidity of cellular membranes. In addition, an association between habitual intake of dietary cholesterol and fasting glucose level was observed in a cross-sectional population survey [188]. This association could partly be explained by an association with saturated fat intake, but effects of cholesterol feeding on glucose levels have also been shown in an experiment with calves [223], as well as in a human intervention study [124]. This requires additional attention in the future.

Dietary Protein

To date no epidemiological data have shown an independent association between protein intake and glucose intolerance. This may be partly due to the strong association of protein intake with the intake of other nutrients, such as saturated fatty acids (for protein of animal origin) or carbohydrates and fiber (for protein of vegetable origin). Vegetable protein intake was indeed related to body fat percentage among obese middle-aged men [162], suggesting a possible effect on glucose metabolism.

Experimental studies have shown that dietary protein, and especially some amino acids such as arginine, leucine and phenylalanine, can stimulate beta cell function [224]. According to the hyperinsulinemia-insulin resistance hypothesis, this could potentially reduce glucose tolerance (fig. 1). However, in epidemiological studies amino acids have not yet been separately investigated. It must be noted that protein recommendations are certainly important in diabetic diets, especially regarding the risk of renal failure complications [225, 226].

Alcohol

Regarding alcohol use it is important to consider the acute and chronic effects separately. These effects may differ; especially in diabetic patients alcohol use may, e.g., result in acute hypoglycemia [227].

The role of habitual alcohol intake on glucose metabolism and the development of diabetes has been investigated only in a limited number of studies. In a cross-sectional survey within the Kaiser-Permanente Medical Care Program an increase in postload glucose levels was noticed with increasing alcohol consumption, but among subjects using more than 9 drinks per day lower glucose levels were observed [228]. In a prospective study on French middle-aged men, liver function, an indicator of alcohol abuse, was an independent predictor of the 4-year diabetes risk [94]. In contrast, in several other prospective studies no association between alcohol use and diabetes incidence was observed [102, 229]. Investigators from the Rancho Bernardo Study, however, recently reported an increased risk for diabetes mellitus with increasing alcohol intake in the obese men within their study population [230]. In some of the other population studies cited above the proportion of heavy drinkers may have been too low to detect an increased risk. In addition, confounding by BMI, fat distribution and smoking habits is an important issue. From these contradictory results a definite conclusion about the role of alcohol use cannot yet be drawn.

Micronutrients

Besides the energy-supplying nutrients, minerals, trace elements and vitamins are involved in glucose metabolism. Evidence mainly originates from animal experiments and intervention studies among diabetic patients [231]. Epidemiological evidence for a role of these micronutrients in the etiology of NIDDM is scarce. Studies on this issue are hampered by the lack of information of these nutrients in food tables. Investigations using parameters of body status, biomarkers of exposure, are therefore preferred. However, such studies have not yet been reported. Likely candidates for a role in the etiology of NIDDM are chromium and its biological active form, the glucose tolerance factor, magnesium, and vitamin B_1 and B_6 [231–233]. Since these nutrients occur in foods such as liver, wheat and meat, future studies on dietary intake involving these foods should, therefore, also take the associated intake of micronutrients into account.

Conclusion

From epidemiological studies of various design, it can be concluded that obesity is involved in glucose metabolism and affects the risk of diabetes mellitus. A comparison of the results from prospective studies indicates that a continuous risk relation exists, also reflected by associations with glucose levels among nondiabetic populations. From the attributable proportions it can be estimated that prevention of overweight, as indicated by BMI ≥ 25 kg/m^2, may result in a reduction of 10–60% of the incidence, with an intermediate value of about 30%. However, despite this theoretical potential, it is clear that other factors also play a role. Besides general obesity the fat distribution over the body is of importance as a determinant of glucose metabolism and diabetes, and several etiologic mechanisms have been suggested. For preventive purposes it seems therefore relevant to investigate whether fat distribution can be affected by changes in lifestyle and environmental factors, and several studies in this area were initiated recently [234]. Apart from energy intake and increased physical activity, smoking, alcohol use and psychological stress have been suggested to be candidates for this purpose, but clear evidence is still lacking.

Independently of obesity, physical exercise has also been observed to have a beneficial effect on glucose metabolism. Due to methodological problems epidemiological evidence is yet scarce. For preventive purposes it can therefore be recommended to consider energy intake, physical activity and obesity as a disorder of energy balance, and to focus on all three components jointly.

The second objective of this review was to a evaluate the role of specific dietary factors in the etiology of glucose intolerance. Although few epidemiological studies have addressed this issue, the results now suggest that water-soluble fiber has a beneficial effect. Concerning carbohydrates and especially simple sugars the results are conflicting. However, the deleterious effects which were previously suggested may have been overestimated. Future epidemiological studies including information on insulin levels will provide further insight.

Dietary fatty acids are also shown to be involved in the onset of abnormalities in glucose metabolism, possibly by affecting cellular membranes and the closely associated lipid metabolism. The epidemiological results indicate associations similar to those known for serum total cholesterol: detrimental effects of saturated fatty acids and potential beneficial impacts of monounsaturated and ω3 polyunsaturated fatty acids were reported. These findings are relevant, not only with respect to the scientific knowledge of the etiology of glucose intolerance and NIDDM, but also because of their agreement with current dietary recommendations for cardiovascular diseases [235]. Thus, if the current preventive policy regarding cardiovascular diseases is implemented and continued, this review suggests that beneficial effects on rates of NIDDM can also be expected.

Acknowledgments

I would like to thank Prof. D. Kromhout for his valuable contributions to the manuscript, and Ms. M.D.A.F. Hoffmans, MSc, for her helpful comments. The financial support from The Netherlands Organization for Scientific Research is gratefully acknowledged.

References

1   West KM: Epidemiology of Diabetes and Its Vascular Lesion. New York, Elsevier, 1978.
2   World Health Organization: Diabetes mellitus. Report of a WHO Study Group. WHO Technical Report Series 727. Geneva, WHO, 1985.
3   Jarret RJ, Keen H, Fuller JH, et al: Worsening to diabetes in men with impaired glucose tolerance ('borderline diabetes'). Diabetologia 1979;16:25–30.
4   Kadowaki T, Miyake Y, Hagura R, et al: Risk factors for worsening to diabetes in subjects with impaired glucose tolerance. Diabetologia 1984;26:44–49.
5   Saad MF, Knowler WC, Pettitt DJ, et al: A two-step model for development of non-insulin-dependent diabetes. Am J Med 1991;90:229–235.
6   Olefsky JM: Pathogenesis of insulin resistance and hyperglycemia in non-insulin-dependent diabetes mellitus. Am J Med 1985;79(suppl 3B):1–7.
7   Reaven GM: Role of insulin resistance in human disease. Diabetes 1988;37:1595–1607.

8   Lillioja S, Mott DM, Howard BV, et al: Impaired glucose tolerance as a disorder of insulin action: Longitudinal and cross-sectional studies in Pima Indians. N Engl J Med 1988;318:1217–1239.

9   Haffner SM, Stern MP, Hazuda HP, et al: Increased insulin concentrations in non-diabetic offspring of diabetic parents. N Engl J Med 1988;20:1297–1301.

10 Saad MF, Knowler WC, Pettitt DJ, et al: Sequential changes in serum insulin concentration during development of non-insulin-dependent diabetes. Lancet 1989;i: 1356–1359.

11 Eriksson J, Franssila-Kallunki A, Ekstrand A, et al: Early metabolic defects in persons at increased risk for non-insulin-dependent diabetes mellitus. N Engl J Med 1989;321:37–43.

12 Warram JH, Martin BC, Krolewski AS, et al: Slow glucose removal rate and hyper-insulinemia precede the development of type II diabetes in the offspring of diabetic parents. Ann Intern Med 1990;113:909–915.

13 Porte D Jr: β-Cells in type II diabetes mellitus. Diabetes 1991;40:166–180.

14 Zimmet P: Non-insulin-dependent (type 2) diabetes mellitus: Does it really exist? Diabetic Med 1989;6:728–735.

15 O'Rahilly S, Turner RC, Matthews DR: Impaired pulsatile secretion of insulin in relatives of patients with non-insulin-dependent diabetes. N Engl J Med 1988;318: 1225–1230.

16 Brosseau JD, Eelkema RC, Crawford AC, et al: Diabetes among the three affiliated tribes: Correlation with degree of Indian inheritance. Am J Publ Health 1979;69: 1277–1278.

17 Serjeantson SW, Owerbach D, Zimmet P, et al: Genetics of diabetes in Nauru: Effects of foreign admixture, HLA antigens and the insulin-gene-linked polymorphism. Diabetologia 1983;25:13–17.

18 Chakraborty R, Ferrell RE, Stern MP, et al: Relationship of prevalence of non-insulin-dependent diabetes mellitus to Amerindian admixture in the Mexican Americans in San Antonio, Texas. Genet Epidemiol 1986;3:435–454.

19 Knowler WC, Williams RC, Pettitt DJ, et al: Gm[3; 5, 13, 14] type 2 diabetes mellitus: An association in American Indians with genetic admixture. Am J Hum Genet 1988;43: 520–526.

20 Knobberling J: Studies on the genetic heterogeneity of diabetes mellitus. Diabetologia 1971;7:46–49.

21 Knowler WC, Pettitt DJ, Savage PJ, et al: Diabetes incidence in Pima Indians: Contributions of obesity and parental diabetes. Am J Epidemiol 1981;113:144–156.

22 Beaty TH, Neel JV, Fajans SS: Identifying risk factors for diabetes in first degree relatives of non-insulin dependent diabetic patients. Am J Epidemiol 1982;115: 380–397.

23 Morris RD, Rimm DL, Hartz AJ, et al: Obesity and heredity in the etiology of non-insulin-dependent diabetes mellitus in 32,662 adult white women. Am J Epidemiol 1989;130:112–121.

24 Colditz GA, Willett WC, Stampfer MJ, et al: Weight as a risk factor for clinical diabetes in women. Am J Epidemiol 1990;132:501–513.

25 Barnett AH, Eff C, Leslie RDG, et al: Diabetes in identical twins: A study of 200 pairs. Diabetologia 1981;20:87–93.

26 Newman B, Selby JV, King M-C, et al: Concordance for type 2 (non-insulin-dependent) diabetes mellitus in male twins. Diabetologia 1987;30:763–768.

27 Vogel F, Motoulsky AG: Human Genetics. Problems and Approaches. Berlin, Springer, 1985, pp 156–164.

28 O'Rahilly S, Wainscoat JS, Turner RC: Type 2 (non-insulin-dependent) diabetes mellitus: New genetics for old nightmares. Diabetologia 1988;31:407–414.

29 Cook JTE, Patel PP, Clark A, et al: Non-linkage of the islet amyloid polypeptide gene with type 2 (non-insulin-dependent) diabetes mellitus. Diabetologia 1991;34:103–108.

30 Davidson MB: The effect of aging on carbohydrate metabolism: A review of the English literature and a practical approach to the diagnosis of diabetes mellitus in the elderly. Metabolism 1979;28:688–705.

31 DeFronzo RA: Glucose intolerance and aging. Diabetes Care 1981;4:493–501.

32 Zavaroni I, Dall'Aglio E, Bruschi F, et al: Effect of age and environmental factors on glucose tolerance and insulin secretion in a worker population. J Am Geriatr Soc 1986;34:271–275.

32 Wang JT, Ho LT, Tang KT, et al: Effect of habitual physical activity on age-related glucose intolerance. J Am Geriatr Soc 1989;37:203–209.

34 Tuomilehto J, Wolf E: Primary prevention of diabetes mellitus. Diabetes Care 1987;10:238–248.

35 Jarrett RJ: Epidemiology and public health aspects of non-insulin-dependent diabetes mellitus. Epidemiol Rev 1989;11:151–171.

36 Stunkard AJ, Harris JR, Pedersen NL, et al: The body-mass index of twins who have been reared apart. N Engl J Med 1990;322:1483–1487.

37 Bouchard C, Tremblay A, Després J-P, et al: The response to long-term overfeeding in identical twins. N Engl J Med 1990;322:1477–1482.

38 Newman B, Selby JV, Quesenberry CP, et al: Nongenetic influences of obesity and other cardiovascular disease risk factors: An analysis of identical twins. Am J Epidemiol 1990;132:767.

39 Danforth E: Diet and obesity. Am J Clin Nutr 1985;41:1132–1145.

40 Bray GA: Obesity – A disease of nutrient or energy balance? Nutr Rev 1987;45:33–43.

41 Kromhout D, Saris WHM, Horst CH: Energy intake, energy expenditure, and smoking in relation to body fatness: The Zutphen Study. Am J Clin Nutr 1988;4:668–674.

42 Mann JI, Houston AC: The aetiology of non-insulin dependent diabetes mellitus; in Mann JI, Pyörälä K, Teuscher A (eds): Diabetes in Epidemiological Perspective. London, Churchill Livingstone, 1983.

43 Bantle JP, Laine DC, CAstle GW, et al: Postprandial glucose and insulin responses to meals containing different carbohydrates in normal and diabetic subjects. N Engl J Med 1983;309:7–12.

44 Jenkins DJA, Wolever TMS, Jenkins AL: Starchy foods and glycemic index. Diabetes Care 1988;11:149–159.

45 Himsworth HP: The dietetic factor determining the glucose tolerance and sensitivity to insulin of healthy men. Clin Sci 1935;2:67–94.

46 Keys A: Seven countries: A multivariate analysis of death and coronary heart disease. Cambridge, Harvard University Press, 1980.

47   Kromhout D, De Lezenne Coulander C: Diet, prevalence and 10 year mortality from coronary heart disease in 871 middle-aged men (The Zutphen Study). Am J Epidemiol 1984;119:733–741.

48   Himsworth HP: Diet and the incidence of diabetes mellitus. Clin Sci 1935;2:117–148.

49   Willett W: Nutritional Epidemiology. New York, Oxford University Press, 1990.

50   West KM, Kalbfleisch JM: Influence of nutritional factors on prevalence of diabetes. Diabetes 1971;20:99–108.

51   Prior IAM, Davidson F: The epidemiology of diabetes in Polynesians and Europeans in New Zealand and the Pacific. N Z Med J 1966;20:375–383.

52   King H, Zimmet P, Raper LR, et al: Risk factors for diabetes in three Pacific populations. Am J Epidemiol 1984;119:396–409.

53   Russell-Jones DL, Hoskins P, Kearney E, Morris R, et al: Rural/urban differences of diabetes – Impaired glucose tolerance, hypertension, obesity, glycosylated haemoglobin, nutritional proteins, fasting cholesterol and apolipoproteins in Fijian Melanesians over 40. Q J Med 1990;273:75–81.

54   Cohen AM: Prevalence of diabetes among different ethnic Jewish groups in Israel. Metabolism 1986;10:50–58.

55   Stern MP, Rosenthal M, Haffner SM, et al: Sex differences in the effects of sociocultural status on diabetes and cardiovascular risk factors in Mexican Americans: The San Antonio Heart Study. Am J Epidemiol 1984;120:834–851.

56   Fujimoto WY, Bergstrom RW, Newell-Morris L, et al: Nature and nurture in the etiology of type 2 diabetes mellitus in Japanese Americans. Diabetes Metab Rev 1989;5:607–625.

57   Kawate R, Yamakido M, Nishimoto Y, et al: Diabetes mellitus and its complications in Japanese migrants on the island of Hawaii: Diabetes Care 1979;2:161–170.

58   Mather HM, Keen H: The Southall Diabetes Survey: Prevalence of known diabetes in Asians and Europeans. Br Med J 1985;291:58.

59   Otsbye T, Welby TJ, Prior IAM, et al: Type 2 (non-insulin-dependent) diabetes mellitus, migration and westernisation: The Tokelau Island Migrant Study. Diabetologia 1989;32:585–590.

60   Himsworth HP, Marshall EM: The diet of diabetics prior to the onset of disease. Clin Sci 1935;2:95–115.

61   Harris MI, Hadden WC, Knowler WC, et al: Prevalence of diabetes and impaired glucose tolerance and plasma glucose levels in U.S. population aged 20–74 years. Diabetes 1987;36:523–534.

62   Baird JD: DIet and the development of clinial diabetes. Acta Diabetol Lat 1972; 9(suppl 1):621–639.

63   Kannel WB, Gordon T, Castelli WP: Obesity, lipids, and glucose intolerance: The Framingham Study. Am J Clin Nutr 1979;32:1238–1245.

64   Bonham GS, Brock DB: The relationship of diabetes with race, sex, and obesity. Am J Clin Nutr 1985;41:776–783.

65   Tuomilehto J, Nissinen A, Kivelä S-L, et al: Prevalence of diabetes mellitus in elderly men aged 65 to 84 years in eastern and western Finland. Diabetologia 1986; 29:611–615.

66   Chen MK, Lowenstein FW: Epidemiology of factors related to self-reported diabetes among adults. Am J Prev Med 1986;2:14–19.

67   Seidell JC, De Groot CPMG, van Sonsbeek JLA, et al: Associations of moderate and severe overweight with self reported illness and medical consumption in Dutch adults. Am J Public Health 1986;76:264–269.

68   Ohlson LO, Larsson B, Eriksson H, et al: Diabetes mellitus in Swedish middle-aged men: The study of men born in 1913 and 1923. Diabetologia 1987;30:386–393.

69   Hartz AJ, Rupley DC, Kalhoff RD, et al: Relationship of obesity to diabetes: Influence of obesity level and body fat distribution. Prev Med 1983;351–357.

70   Laasko M, Barrett-Connor E: Asymptomatic hyperglycemia is associated with lipid and lipoprotein changes favoring atherosclerosis. Arteriosclerosis 1989;9:665–672.

71   Burchfiel CM, Hamman RF, Marshall JA, et al: Cardiovascular risk factors and impaired glucose tolerance: The San Luis Valley Diabetes Study. Am J Epidemiol 1990;131:57–70.

72   Newell-Morris LL, Treder RP, Shuman WP, et al: Fatness, fat distribution, and glucose tolerance in second-generation Japanese American (Nisei) men. Am J Clin Nutr 1989;50:9–18.

73   Barrett-Connor E: Factors associated with the distribution of fasting plasma glucose in an adult community. Am J Epidemiol 1980;112:518–523.

74   Feskens EJM, Kromhout D: Effects of body fat and its development over a ten-year period on glucose tolerance in euglycaemic men: The Zutphen Study. Int J Epidemiol 1989;18:368–373.

75   Olefsky JM, Kolterman OG: Mechanisms of insulin resistance in obesity and non-insulin dependent (type II) diabetes. Am J Med 1981;70:151–168.

76   Laakso M, Pyörälä K, Voutilainen E, et al: Plasma insulin and serum lipids and lipoproteins in middle-aged non-insulin-dependent diabetic and non-diabetic subjects. Am J Epidemiol 1987;125:611–621.

77   Lichtenstein MJ, Yarnell JWG, Elwood PC, et al: Sex hormones, insulin, lipids, and prevalent ischemic heart disease. Am J Epidemiol 1987;126:647–657.

78   Donahue RP, Orchard TJ, Becker DJ, et al: Physical activity, insulin sensitivity, and the lipoprotein profile in young adults: The Beaver County Study. Am J Epidemiol 1988;127:95–103.

79   Wing RR, Bunker CH, Kuller LH, et al: Insulin, body mass index, and cardiovascular risk factors in premenopausal women. Arteriosclerosis 1989;9:479–484.

80   Seidell JC, Cigolini M, Charzewska J, et al: Fat distribution in European women: A comparison of anthropometric measurements in relation to cardiovascular risk factors. Int J Epidemiol 1990;19:303–308.

81   Manolio TA, Savage PJ, Burke GL, et al: Association of fasting insulin with blood pressure and lipids in young adults: The CARDIA Study. Arteriosclerosis 1990;10:430–436.

82   Montoye HJ, Block WD, Metzner H, et al: Habitual physical activity and glucose tolerance: Males age 16–64 in a total community. Diabetes 1977;26:172–176.

83   Sobolski J, Kornitzer M, De Backer G, et al: Protection against ischemic heart disease in the Belgian Physical Fitness Study: Physical fitness rather than physical activity? Am J Epidemiol 1987;125:601–610.

84   Ekelund L-G, Haskell WL, Johnson JL, et al: Physical finess as a predictor of car-

diovascular mortality in asymptomatic North American men: The Lipids Research Clinics Mortality Follow-Up Study. N Engl J Med 1988;319:1379–1384.

85 Berntorp K, Lindgärde F, Malmquist J: High and low insulin responders: Relations to oral glucose tolerance, insulin secretion and physical fitness. Acta Med Scand 1984;216:111–117.

86 Sopko G, Jacobs DR, Raylor HL: Dietary measures of physical activity. Am J Epidemiol 1984;120:900–911.

87 Slattery ML, Jacobs DR, Nichaman MZ: An assessment of caloric intake as an indicator of physical activity. Prev Med 1989;18:444–451.

88 Romieu I, Willett WC, Stampfer MJ, et al: Energy intake and other derterminants of relative weight. Am J Clin Nutr 1988;47:406–412.

89 Keen H, Thomas BJ, Jarrett RJ, et al: Nutrient intake, adiposity, and diabetes. Br Med J 1979;i:655–658.

90 Thomas BJ, Jarrett RJ, Keen H, et al: Relation of habitual diet to fasting plasma insulin concentration and the insulin response to oral glucose. Hum Nutr 1982;36C: 49–56.

91 Westlund K, Nicolaysen R: Ten-year mortality and morbidity related to serum cholesterol: A follow-up of 3,751 men aged 40–49. Scand J Clin Lab Invest 1972; 30(suppl 127):3–24.

92 Pfaffenbarger RS Jr, Wing AL: Chronic disease in former college students. XII. Early precursors of adult-onset diabetes mellitus. Am J Epidemiol 1973;97:314–323.

93 Medalie JH, Papier CM, Goldbourt U, et al: Major factors in the development of diabetes mellitus in 10,000 men. Arch Intern Med 1975;135:811–817.

94 Papoz L, Eschwege E, Warnet J-M, et al: Incidence and risk factors of diabetes in the Paris Protective Study (GREA); in Eschwege E (ed): Advances in Diabetes Epidemiology. Amsterdam, Elsevier, 1982, pp 113–122.

95 Butler WJ, Ostrander LD Jr, Carman WJ, et al: Diabetes mellitus in Tecumseh, Michigan: Prevalence, incidence, and associated conditions. Am J Epidemiol 1982; 116:971–980.

96 Balkau B, King H, Zimmet P, et al: Factors associated with the development of diabetes in the Micronesian population of Nauru. Am J Epidemiol 1985;122:594–605.

97 Ohlson LO, Larsson B, Björntorp P, et al: Risk factors for type 2 (non-insulin-dependent) diabetes mellitus: Thirteen and one-half years of follow-up of the participants in a study of Swedish men born in 1913. Diabetologia 1988;31:798–805.

98 Wilson PWF, Anderson KM, Kannel WB: Epidemiology of diabetes mellitus in the elderly: The Framington Study. Am J Med 1986;80(suppl 5A):3–9.

99 Modan M, Karasik A, Halkin H, et al: Effect of past and concurrent body mass index on prevalence of glucose intolerance and type 2 (non-insulin-dependent) diabetes and on insulin response: The Israel study of glucose intolerance, obesity and hypertension. Diabetologia 1986;29:82–89.

100 Seidell JC, Bakx KC, van de Hooge HJM, et al: Overweight and chronic illness – A retrospective cohort study, with a follow-up of 6–17 years, in men and women of initially 20–50 years of age. J Chronic Dis 1986;39:585–593.

101 Lundgren H, Bengtsson C, Blohmé G, et al: Dietary habits and incidence of noninsulin-dependent diabetes mellitus in a population of women in Gothenburg, Sweden. Am J Clin Nutr 1989;49:708–712.

102 Feskens EJM, Kromhout D: Cardiovascular risk factors and the 25-year incidence of diabetes mellitus: The Zutphen Study. Am J Epidemiol 1989;130:1101–1108.

103 McPhillips JB, Barrett-Connor E, Wingard DL: Cardiovascular disease risk factors prior to the diagnosis of impaired glucose tolerance and non-insulin-dependent diabetes mellitus in a community of older adults. Am J Epidemiol 1990;131:443–453.

104 Haffner SM, Stern MP, Mitchell BD, et al: Incidence of type II diabetes in Mexican Americans predicted by fasting insulin and glucose levels, obesity, and body fat distribution. Diabetes 1990;39:283–288.

105 Hedges LV, Olkin I: Statistical Methods for Meta-Analysis. Orlando, Academic Press, 1985.

106 Rothman KJ: Modern Epidemiology. Boston, Little, Brown, 1986.

107 Greenland S, Robins J: Conceptual problems in the definition and interpretation of attributable fractions. Am J Epidemiol 1988;128:1185–1197.

108 Feskens EJM, Bowles CH, Kromhout D: Carbohydrate intake and body mass index in relation to the risk of glucose intolerance in an elderly population. Am J Clin Nutr 1991;54:136–140.

109 Keen H, Jarrett RJ, McCartney P: The ten year follow-up of the Bedford survey (1962–1972): Glucose tolerance and diabetes. Diabetologia 1982;22:73–78.

110 Saad MF, Knowler WC, Pettitt D, et al: The natural history of impaired glucose tolerance in the Pima Indians. N Engl J Med 1988;319:150–156.

111 Barrett-Connor E: Epidemiology, obesity, and non-insulin-dependent diabetes mellitus. Epidemiol Rev 1989;11:172–181.

112 Everhart JE, Pettitt DJ, Slaine KR, et al: Duration of obesity is a risk factor for non-insulin-dependent diabetes mellitus (abstract). Am J Epidemiol 1986;124:525.

113 Medalie JH, Papier C, Herman JB, et al: Diabetes mellitus among 10,000 adult men. I. Five-year incidence and associated variables. Isr J Med Sci 1974;10:681–697.

114 Tell GS, Vellar OD: Physical fitness, physical activity, and cardiovascular disease risk factors in adolescents: The Oslo Youth Study. Prev Med 1988;17:12–24.

115 Kaye SA, Folsom AR, Sprafka JM, et al: Increased incidence of diabetes mellitus in relation to abdominal adiposity in older women. J Clin Epidemiol 1991;44:329–334.

116 Helmrich SP, Ragland DR, Leung RW, et al: Physical activity and reduced occurrence of non-insulin-dependent diabetes mellitus. N Engl J Med 1991;325:147–152.

117 Ashley FW, Kannel WB: Relation of weight change to changes in atherogenic traits: The Framingham Study. J Chronic Dis 1974;27:103–114.

118 Noppa H: Body weight change in relation to incidence of ischemic heart disease and change in risk factors for ischemic heart disease. Am J Epidemiol 1980;111:693–704.

119 Borkan GA, Sparrow D, Wisniewski C, et al: Body weight and coronary disease risk: Patterns of risk factor change associated with long-term weight change. Am J Epidemiol 1986;124:410–419.

120 Feskens EJM, Bowles CH, Kromhout D: A longitudinal study on glucose tolerance and other cardiovascular risk factors: Associations within an elderly population. J Clin Epidemiol (in press).

121 Bennett PH: Impaired glucose tolerance: A target for intervention? Arteriosclerosis 1985;32:864–869.

122 Sartor G, Schersten B, Carlstrom S, et al: Ten-year follow-up of subjects with impaired glucose tolerance: Prevention of diabetes by tolbutamide and diet regulation. Diabetes 1980;29:41–49.

123 Farinaro E, Stamler J, Upton J, et al: Plasma glucose levels: Long-term effect of diet in the Chicago Coronary Prevention Evaluation Program. Ann Intern Med 1977;86: 147–154.

124 Coon PJ, Bleecker ER, Drinkwater DT, et al: Effect of body composition and exercise capacity on glucose tolerance, insulin, and lipoprotein lipids in healthy older men: A cross-sectional and longitudinal intervention study. Metabolism 1989;38: 1201–1209.

125 Tremblay A, Nadeau A, Després J-P, et al: Long-term exercise training with constant energy intake. 2. Effect on glucose metabolism and resting energy expenditure. Int J Obes 1990;14:75–84.

126 Rauramaa R: Relationship of physical activity, glucose tolerance, and weight management. Prev Med 1984;13:37–46.

127 Hughes TA, Gwynne JT, Switzer BR, et al: Effects of caloric restriction and weight loss on glycemic control, insulin release and resistance, and atherosclerotic risk in obese patients with type II diabetes mellitus. Am J Med 1984;77:7–17.

128 Krotkiewski M, Lonnroth P, Mandroukas K, et al: The effects of physical training on insulin secretion and effectiveness and on glucose metabolism in obesity and type 2 (non-insulin-dependent) diabetes mellitus. Diabetologia 1985;28:881–890.

129 Uusitupa MIJ, Laakso M, Sarlund H, et al: Effects of a very-low-calorie diet on metabolic control and cardiovascular risk factors in the treatment of obese non-insulin-dependent diabetics. Am J Clin Nutr 1990;51:768–773.

130 American Diabetes Association: Nutritional recommendations and principles for individuals with diabetes mellitus: 1986. Diabetes Care 1987;10:126–132.

131 Vague J: The degree of masculine differentiation of obesities: A factor determining predisposition to diabetes, atherosclerosis, gout, and uric calculous disease. Am J Clin Nutr 1956;4:20–34.

132 Feldman R, Sender AJ, Siegelaub AB: Difference in diabetic and nondiabetic fat distribution patterns by skinfold measurements. Diabetes 1969;18:478–486.

133 Joos SK, Mueller WH, Hanis CL, et al: Diabetes Alert Study: Weight history and upper body obesity in diabetic and non-diabetic Mexican American adults. Ann Hum Biol 1984;11:167–171.

134 Harlan LC, Harlan WR, Landis JR, et al: Factors associated with glucose tolerance in U.S. adults. Am J Epidemiol 1987;126:674–684.

135 Freedman DS, Srinivasan SR, Burke GL, et al: Relation of body fat distribution to hyperinsulinemia in children and adolescents: The Bogalusa Heart Study. Am J Clin Nutr 1987;46:403–410.

136 Young TK, Sevenhuysen GP, Ling N, et al: Determinants of plasma glucose level and diabetic status in a northern Canadian Indian population. Can Med Assoc J 1990;142:821–830.

137 Bray GA, Greenway FL, Molitch ME, et al: Use of anthropometric measures to assess weight loss. Am J Clin Nutr 1978;31:769–773.

138 Sparrow D, Borkan GA, Gerzof SG, et al: Relationship of fat distribution to glucose tolerance: Results of computed tomography in male participants of the Normative Aging Study. Diabetes 1986;35:411–415.

139 Seidell JC, Björntorp P, Sjöström L, et al: Regional distribution of muscle and fat mass in men – New insights into the risk of abdominal obesity using computed tomography. Int J Obes 1989;13:289–303.

140 Björntorp P: The association between obesity, adipose tissue distribution and disease. Acta Med Scand 1988(suppl 723);121–134.

141 Kissebah AH, Vydelingum N, Murray R, et al: Relation of body fat distribution to metabolic complications of obesity. J Clin Endocrinol Metab 1982;54:254–260.

142 Krotkiewski M, Björntorp P, Sjöström L, et al: Impact of obesity on metabolism in men and women: Importance of regional adipose tissue distribution. J Clin Invest 1983;72:1150–1162.

143 Kalhoff RK, Hartz AH, Rupley D, et al: Relationship of body fat distribution to blood pressure, carbohydrate tolerance, and plasma lipids in healthy obese women. J Lab Clin Med 1983;102:621–627.

144 Evans DJ, Hoffmann RG, Kalkhoff RK, et al: Relationship of body fat topography to insulin sensitivity and metabolic profiles in premenopausal women. Metabolism 1984;33:68–75.

145 Ohlson LO, Larsson B, Svärssud K, et al: The influence of body fat distribution on the incidence of diabetes mellitus: 13.5 years of follow-up of the participants in the study of men born in 1913. Diabetes 1985;34:1055–1058.

146 Freedman DS, Rimm A: The relation of body fat distribution, as assessed by six grith measurenments, to diabetes mellitus in women. Am J Publ Health 1989;79: 715–720.

147 Seidell JC, Cigolini M, Charzewska J, et al: Androgenicity in relation to body fat distribution and metabolism in 38-year-old women: The European Fat Distribution Study. J Clin Epidemiol 1990;43:21–34.

148 Van Noord PA, Seidell JC, den Tonkelaar I, et al: The relationship between fat distribution and some chronic diseases in 11,825 women participating in the DOM project. Int J Epidemiol 1990;19:564–570.

149 McKeigue PM, Shah B, Marmot MG: Relation of central obesity and insulin resistance with high diabetes prevalence and cardiovascular risk in South Asians. Lancet 1991;337:382–386.

150 Iso H, Kiyama M, Naito Y, et al: The relation of body fat distribution and body mass with haemoglobin A_{1c}, blood pressure and blood lipids in urban Japanese men. Int J Epidemiol 1991;20:88–94.

151 Haffner S, Stern MP, Hazuda H, et al: Do upper-body and centralized adiposity measure different aspects of regional body-fat distribution? Diabetes 1987;36:43–51.

152 Després J-P, Nadeau A, Tremblay A, et al: Role of deep abdominal fat in the association between regional adipose tissue distribution and glucose tolerance in obese women. Diabetes 1989;38:304–309.

153 Bergstrom RW, Newell-Morris LL, Leonetti DL, et al: Association of elevated fasting C-peptide level and increased intra-abdominal fat distribution with development of NIDDM in Japanese-American men. Diabetes 1990;39:104–111.

154 Kvist H, Chowdhury C, Grengard U, et al: Total and visceral adipose-tissue volumes derived from measurements with computed tomography in adult men and women: Predictive equations. Am J Clin Nutr 1988;48:1351–1361.

155 Kissebah AH, Peiris AN: Biology of regional body fat distribution: Relationship to non-insulin-dependent diabetes mellitus. Diabetes Metab Rev 1989;5:83–109.

156 DeFronzo RA, Ferrannini E, Koivisto V: New concepts in the pathogenesis and treatment of noninsulin-dependent diabetes mellitus. Am J Med 1983;79(suppl 3B): 52–81.

157 Randle PJ, Garland PB, Hales CN, et al: The glucose-fatty acid cycle: Its role in insulin sensitivity and the metabolic disturbances of diabetes mellitus. Lancet 1963; ii:185–189.

158 Peiris AN, Sothman MS, Hofman RG, et al: Adiposity, fat distribution and cardio-vascular risk. Ann Intern Med 1989;110:867–872.

159 Neel JV: Diabetes mellitus: A 'thrifty' genotype rendered detrimental by 'progress'? Am J Hum Genet 1962;14:353–362.

160 Wendorf M, Goldfine ID: Archaeology of NIDDM: Excavation of the 'thrifty' geno-type. Diabetes 1991;40:161–165.

161 Henry RR, Wallace P, Olefsky JM: Effects of weight loss on mechanisms of hyper-glycemia in obese non-insulin-dependent diabetes mellitus. Diabetes 1986;35:990–998.

162 Dreon D, Frey-Hewitt B, Ellsworth N, et al: Dietary fat:carbohydrate ratio and obesity in middle-aged men. Am J Clin Nutr 1987;47:995–1000.

163 Feldberg W, Pyke DA, Stubbs WA: On the origin of non-insulin-dependent diabetes. Lancet 1986;i:1263–1264.

164 Surwit RS, Feinglos MN: Stress and autonomic nervous system in type II diabetes: A hypothesis. Diabetes Care 1988;11:83–85.

165 Barret-Connor E, Khaw K-T: Cigarette smoking and increased central adiposity. Ann Intern Med 1989;111:783–787.

166 Shimokata H, Muller DC, Andres R: Studies in the distribution of body fat. III. Effects of cigarette smoking. JAMA 1989;261:1169–1173.

167 Seidell JC, Cigolini M, Deslypere J-P, et al: Body fat distribution in relation to physical activity and smoking habits in 38-year-old European men. Am J Epidemiol 1991;133:257–265.

168 Bertorp K, Trell E, Thorell J, et al: Relation between plasma insulin and blood glucose in a cross-sectional population study of the oral glucose tolerance test. Acta Endocrinol 1983;102:549–556.

169 Williamson DF, Madans J, Anda RF, et al: Smoking cessation and severity of weight gain in a national cohort. N Engl J Med 1991;324:739–745.

170 Cryer PE, Haymond MW, Santiageo JV, et al: Norepinephrine and epinephrine release and adrenergic mediation of smoking-associated hemodynamic and meta-bolic events. N Engl J Med 1976;295:573–577.

171 Van Barneveld T, Seidell JC, Traag N, et al: Fat distribution and gamma-glutamyl transferase in relation to serum lipids and blood pressure in 38-year old males. Eur J Clin Nutr 1989;43:809–818.

172 Hellerstedt WL, Jeffery RW, Murray DM: The association between alcohol intake and adiposity in the general population. Am J Epidemiol 1990;132:594–611.

173 Haffner SM, Stern MP, Hazuda HP, et al: Upper body and centralized adiposity in Mexican Americans and non-Hispanic whites: Relationship to body mass index and other behavioral and demographic variables. Int J Obes 1986;10:493–502.

174 Vansant G, Den Besten C, Westrate J, et al: Body fat distribution and the prognosis for weight reduction: Preliminary observations. Int J Obes 1988;12:133–140.

175 Mann JI, Truswell AS: Effects of isocaloric exchange of dietary sucrose and starch on fasting serum lipids, postprandial insulin secretion and alimentary lipaemia in human subjects. Br J Nutr 1972;27:395–405.

176 Anderson JW, Herman RH, Zakim D: Effect of high glucose and high sucrose diets on glucose tolerance of normal men. Am J Clin Nutr 1973;26:600–607.

177 Jenkins DJA, Leeds AR, Gassull MA, et al: Decrease in postprandial insulin and glucose concentrations by guar and pectin. Ann Intern Med 1977;86:20–23.

178 Crapo PA, Reaven G, Olefsky J: Postprandial plasma-glucose and -insulin responses to different complex carbohydrates. Diabetes 1977;26:1178–1183.

179 Jenkins DJA, Wolever TMS, Leeds AR, et al: Dietary fibres, fiber analogues, and glucose tolerance: Importance of viscosity. Br Med J 1978;i:1392–1394.

180 Munoz JM, Sandstead HH, Jacob RA: Effects of dietary fiber on glucose tolerance of normal men. Diabetes 1979;28:496–502.

181 Reiser S, Handler HB, Gardner LB, et al: Isocaloric exchange of dietary starch and sucrose in humans. II. Effect of fastsing blood insulin, glucose, and glucagon and on insulin and glucose responses to a sucrose load. Am J Clin Nutr 1979;32:2206–2216.

182 Aro A, Uusitupa M, Voitilanen R, et al: Improved diabetic control and hypocholesterolemic effect induced by long term dietary supplementation with guar gum in type II (non-insulin-dependent diabetes). Diabetologia 1981;21:29–33.

183 Collier G, O'Dea K: The effect of coingestion of fat on the glucose, insulin, and gastric inhibitory polypeptide responses to carbohydrate and protein. Am J Clin Nutr 1983;37:941–944.

184 Brand JC, Colagiuri S, Crossman S, et al: Low-glycemic index foods improve long-term glycemic control in NIDDM. Diabetes Care 1991;14:95–101.

185 Yudkin J: Dietary fat and dietary sugar in relation to ischemic heart disease and diabetes. Lancet 1964;i:4–5.

186 Cleave TL: The Saccharine Disease. Bristol, Wright, 1974, pp 80–96.

187 Trowell HC: Dietary-fiber hypothesis of the etiology of diabetes mellitus. Diabetes 1975;24:762–765.

188 Feskens EJM, Kromhout D: Habitual dietary intake and glucose tolerance in middle-aged euglycaemic men: The Zutphen Study. Int J Epidemiol 1990;19:953–959.

189 Prentice AM, Black AE, Coward WA, et al: High levels of energy expenditure in obese women. Br Med J 1986;292:983–987.

190 Kahn HA, Herman JB, Medalie JH, et al: Factors related to diabetes incidence: A multivariate analysis of two years observation on 10,000 men. J Chronic Dis 1971;23:617–629.

191 Bossetti BM, Kocher LM, Morranz JF, et al: The effects of physiologic amounts of simple sugars on lipoprotein, glucose and insulin levels in normal subjects. Diabetes Care 1984;7:309–312.

192 Wolever TMS: Relationship between dietary fiber content and composition in foods and the glycemic index. Am J Clin Nutr 1990;51:72–75.

193 Ray TK, Mansell KM, Knight LC, et al: Long-term effects of dietary fiber on glucose tolerance and gastric emptying in noninsulin-dependent diabetic patients. Am J Clin Nutr 1983;37:376–381.

194 Schwartz SE, Levine RA, Siongh A, et al: Sustained pectin ingestion delays gastric emptying. Gastroenterology 1982;83:12–17.

195 Bennett PH, Knowler WC, Baird HR, et al: Diet and the development of noninsulin-dependent diabetes mellitus: An epidemiological perspective; in Pozza G et al. (eds): Diet, Diabetes, and Atherosclerosis. New York, Raven Press, 1984, pp 109–119.

196 Sadur CN, Yost TJ, Eckel RH: Fat feeding decreases insulin responsiveness of adipose tissue lipoprotein lipase. Metabolism 1984;33:1043–1047.

197 Chisholm K, O'Dea K: Effect of short-term consumption of a high-fat, low-carbohydrate diet on metabolic control in insulin-deficient diabetic rats. Metabolism 1987; 36:237–243.

198 Snowdon DA, Phillips RL: Does a vegetarian diet reduce the occurrence of diabetes? Am J Public Health 1985;75:507–512.

199 Trevisan M, Krogh V, Freudenheim J, et al: Consumption of olive oil, butter and vegetable oils and coronary heart disease risk factors. JAMA 1990;263:688–692.

200 Pelikánová T, Kohout M, Valek J, et al: Insulin secretion and insulin action related to the serum phospholipid fatty acid pattern in healthy men. Metabolism 1989;38: 188–192.

201 Tsunehara, CH, Leonetti DL, Fujimoto WY: Animal fat and cholesterol intake is high in men with IGT progressing to NIDDM. Diabetes 1991;40:427A.

202 Tsunehara CH, Leonetti DL, Fujimoto WF: Diet of second-generation Japanese-American men with and without non-insulin-dependent diabetes. Am J Clin Nutr 1990;52:731–738.

203 Lardinois CK: The role of omega 3 fatty acids on insulin secretion and insulin sensitivity. Med Hypotheses 1987;24:243–248.

204 Kromann N, Green A: Epidemiological studies in the Upernavik District, Greenland. Acta Med Scand 1980;208:401–406.

205 Mouratoff GJ, Carroll NV, Scot EM: Diabetes mellitus in Athabaskan indians in Alaska. Diabetes 1969;18:29–32.

206 Feskens EJM, Bowles CH, Kromhout D: Inverse association between fish intake and risk of glucose intolerance in normoglycemic elderly men and women. Diabetes Care, 1991;14:935–941.

207 Smith U, Kral J, Björntorp P: Influence of dietary fat and carbohydrate on the metabolism of adipocytes of different size in the rat. Biochim Biophys Acta 1974; 337:278–285.

208 Ginsberg BH, Jabour J, Spector AA: Effect of alterations in membrane lipid unsaturation on the properties of the insulin receptor of Ehrlich ascites cells. Biochim Biophys Acta 1982;690:157–164.

209 Robertson RP: Eicosanoids as pluripotential modulators of pancreatic islet function. Diabetes 1988;37:367–370.

210 Kinsell LW, Walker G, Michels GD, et al: Dietary fats and the diabetic patient. N Engl J Med 1959;261:431–434.

211 Houtsmuller AJ: The role of fat in the treatment of diabetes mellitus; in Vergroesen AJ (ed): The Role of Fats in Human Nutrition. New York, Academic Press, 1975, pp 231–302.

212 Houtsmuller AJ, Van Hal-Ferwerda J, Zahn KJ, et al: Favourable influences of linoleic acid on the progression of diabetic micro- and macroangiopathy. Nutr Metab 1980;24(suppl 1):105–118.

213 Heine RJ, Mulder C, Popp-Snijders C, et al: Linoleic-acid-enriched diet: Long-term effects on serum lipoprotein and apolipoprotein concentrations and insulin sensitivity in noninsulin-dependent diabetic patients. Am J Clin Nutr 1989;49:448–456.

214 Storlien LH, Jenkins AB, Chisholm DJ, et al: Influence of dietary fat composition on development of insulin resistance in rats. Diabetes 1991;40:280–289.

215 Garg A, Bonamone A, Grundy SM, et al: Comparison of a high-carbohydrate diet with a high-monounsaturated-fat diet in patients with non-insulin-dependent diabetes mellitus. N Engl J Med 1988;319:829–834.

216 Storlien LH, Kragen EW, Chisholm DJ, et al: Fish oil prevents insulin resistance induced by high-fat feeding in rats. Science 1987;237:885–888.

217 Woehrle M, Giessler D, Lin Th, et al: The influence of a special fish oil diet on insulitis and on the incidence of diabetes in the BB rat. Diabetologia 1989;32:557A–558A.

218 Waldhäusl W, Ratheiser K, Komjati M, et al: Increase of insulin sensitivity and improvement of intravenous glucose tolerance by fish oil in healthy man; in Chandra RK (ed): Health Effects of Fish and Fish Oils. St. John's, ARTS Biomedical, 1989, pp 171–187.

219 Kromhout D, Bosschieter EB, de Lezenne Coulander C: The inverse relation between fish consumption and 20-year mortality from coronary heart disease. N Engl J Med 1985;312:1205–1209.

220 Phillipson BE, Rothrock DW, Connor WE, et al: Reduction of plasma lipids, lipoproteins, and apoproteins by dietary fish oil in patients with hypertriglyceridemia. N Engl J Med 1985;312:1210–1216.

221 Popp-Snijders C, Schouten JA, Heine RJ, et al: Dietary supplementation of omega-3 polyunsaturated fatty acids improves insulin sensitivity in non-insulin-dependent diabetes. Diabetes Res 1987;4:141–147.

222 Srinivasan SR, Amos C, Albares R, et al: Inflence of serum lipoprotein and carbohydrate metabolism on erythrocyte membrane composition in children: Bogalusa Heart Study. Metabolism 1986;35:466–471.

223 Beynen AC, van Gils LGM: Diurnal patterns of the concentrations of cholesterol, triglycerides, glucose, nonprotein nitrogen and urea in the serum of veal calves fed a milk replacer supplemented with cholesterol. Z Ernährungswiss 1983;22:50–58.

224 Ward WK, Beard JC, Halter JB: Pathophysiology of insulin secretion in non-insulin-dependent diabetes mellitus. Diabetes Care 1984;7:491–502.

225 Nuttall FQ: Diet and the diabetic patient. Diabetes Care 1983;6:197–207.

226 Wylie-Rosett J: Evaluation of protein in dietary management of diabetes mellitus. Diabetes Care 1988;11:143–148.

227 Marks V: Alcohol and carbohydrate metabolism. Clin Endocrinol Metab 1978;7:333–349.

228 Gérard MJ, Klatsky AL, Siegelaub AB, et al: Serum glucose levels and alcohol-consumption habits in a large population. Diabetes 1977;26:780–785.

229 Stampfer MJ, Colditz GA, Willett WC, et al: A prospective study of moderate alcohol drinking and risk of diabetes in women. Am J Epidemiol 1988;128:549–558.
230 Holbrook TL, Barrett-Connor E, Wingard DL: A prospective population-based study of alcohol use and non-insulin-dependent diabetes mellitus. Am J Epidemiol 1990;132:902–909.
231 Mooradian AD, Morley JE: Micronutrient status in diabetes mellitus. Am J Clin Nutr 1987;45:877–895.
232 Boyle E Jr, Mondschein B, Dash HH: Chromium depletion in the pathogenesis of diabetes and atherosclerosis. South Med J 1977;70:1449–1453.
233 Foster H: Diabetes mellitus and low environmental magnesium levels. Lancet 1987; ii:633.
234 Van de Kooy K, Leenen R, Seidell JC, et al: Changes in abdominal fat and diameters with weight loss: A magnetic resonance imaging study. Int J Obes 1991;15(suppl 1): 88.
235 Nutriton Council: Guidelinse for a Healthy Diet. The Hague, Nutrition Council, 1986.

Edith J.M. Feskens, Department of Epidemiology, National Institute of
Public Health and Environmental Protection, PO Box 1,
NL–3720 BA Bilthoven (The Netherlands)

Simopoulos AP (ed): Nutrients in the Control of Metabolic Diseases.
World Rev Nutr Diet. Basel, Karger, 1992, vol 69, pp 40–73

Vitamins and Hypertension[1]

K. Dakshinamurti, K.J. Lal

Department of Biochemistry and Molecular Biology, Faculty of Medicine,
University of Manitoba, Winnipeg, Man., Canada

Contents

Introduction   40
Vitamin B_6   42
    Pyridoxine Deficiency: Animal Model of Hypertension   44
    Characterization of Hypertension Induced by Vitamin B_6 Deficiency   47
Vitamin D   60
Vitamin E   65
Conclusions   66
References   67

Introduction

Hypertension, the sustained elevation of systemic arterial pressure with a systolic pressure over 160 mm Hg and a diastolic pressure greater than 95 mm Hg, is one of the major causes of chronic illness in western and acculturated communities. In western societies, about 20–30% of the adult population have some degree of elevation of blood pressure. The introduction of thiazides and β-blocking drugs ushered a new chapter in the treatment of hypertension with satisfying control of blood pressure with relatively minimal side effects. Asymptomatic hypertensives are consigned to a lifetime of drug treatment. The psychological impact of being a

[1] This work was supported by grants from The Manitoba Heart and Stroke Foundation and The Medical Research Council of Canada.

patient for life is profound. Currently, there is increasing awareness of the adverse effects of therapeutic drugs on the metabolism of lipids and carbohydrates. In view of this there is renewed interest in nondrug treatment of hypertension. It was recognized early that some communities with distinctive life-styles do not have the high incidence of hypertension as in the general population. Vegetarians, in general, have lower blood pressure than omnivore populations. Increased consumption of salt (sodium chloride), sugar, saturated fat and alcohol as well as obesity have been associated with increased incidence of hypertension. On the other hand, increased intakes of dietary fiber, potassium and polyunsaturated fatty acids have variously been suggested to prevent or ameliorate existing moderate hypertension. There is no clear indication whether these dietary manipulations are useful in reducing hypertension and, if so, under what conditions and by which mechanisms.

Hypertension is produced by many factors such as hypersecretion of aldosterone, mineralocorticoids or glucocorticoids, catecholamine-secreting tumors of adrenal medullary or paraganglionic origin, renal disease and narrowing of the renal arteries or of the aorta. It is also associated with toxemia of pregnancy. In over 90% of patients with elevated blood pressure the causative factors have not been recognized yet. This is referred to as essential hypertension. In early stages of essential hypertension there is an exaggerated pressor response to various stimuli, indicating overactivity of the autonomic system. There is much research activity in trying to identify the primary cause of essential hypertension. Various animal models which approximate the clinical findings in humans have been produced for intensive investigation of this progressive disease process. Apart from as yet undetermined genetic factors, other causative factors such as endocrine abnormalities, alterations in the synthesis of various prostanoids and atrial natriuretic factor as well as impairment in the regulation of cell calcium have been implicated.

The contribution of dietary, life-style and environmental factors to the development of hypertension has received much attention. In this context the roles of various minerals and vitamins have been investigated. Vitamin D is involved in calcium homeostasis. Vitamin E is an antioxidant and has a role in maintaining the integrity of cell membrane. As such it is conceivable that abnormalities in the metabolism of these vitamins could lead to impairment in blood pressure regulation. Among the water-soluble vitamins, only vitamin B_6 (pyridoxine) seems to be involved in the mechanisms regulating blood pressure. This is ascribed to the role of pyridoxal phosphate as the cofactor of the decarboxylases synthesizing the putative neurotransmitters. This review will focus on the mechanisms of action of vitamin B_6, vitamin D and vitamin E as the only vitamins implicated in blood pressure regulation.

Vitamin B_6

Various reports have indicated a relationship between vitamin B_6 status and hypertension in pregnant women and women on anovulatory steroids [1, 2]. Klieger et al. [3] have reported that the toxemic placenta is markedly deficient in pyridoxal phosphate. The lack of demonstrable therapeutic value of vitamin B_6 in toxemia has been ascribed to the low pyridoxine kinase activity in the toxemic placenta. As suggested by Klieger et al. [3], the decrease in the conversion of pyridoxine to pyridoxal phosphate due to the decrease in the activity of the Zn^{2+} or Mg^{2+}-requiring pyridoxal kinase in women prone to the preeclamptic syndrome is a possibility. Zinc supplements during pregnancy reduced the incidence of pregnancy-induced hypertension [4]. The EEG of an eclamptic patient who had seizures was returned to normal following administration of Mg^{2+} and pyridoxine [Brophy, pers. communication]. Hypomagnesemia is also associated with preeclampsia [5]. Seizures associated with pregnancy-induced hypertension are prevented by the administration of magnesium alone [6] or in association with pyridoxine. This indicates the possible activation of pyridoxal kinase resulting in increased in vivo concentration of pyridoxal phosphate. Even in normal pregnancy there is a gradual decrease in serum pyridoxal phosphate which is very significant in the third trimester. This is considerably exaggerated in the preeclamptic state.

Brophy [7] has reported decreased levels of plasma γ-aminobutyric acid (GABA) in zinc-deficient eclamptics. This might again be related to the decreased formation of pyridoxal phosphate, the cofactor of the GABA-synthesizing enzyme glutamic acid decarboxylase. Many reports also suggest an increase in the frequency of hypertensives among chronic alcoholics [8] and diabetics [9]. Decreases in the concentration of plasma pyridoxal phosphate have been reported in both these conditions [10, 11]. Thus, many factors confound the underlying vitamin B_6 status of these individuals. Various clinical reports [12, 13] indicate a correlation between hypothyroidism and hypertension. Saito et al. [13] reported that the hypothyroid state accelerated the age-related increase in blood pressure. On

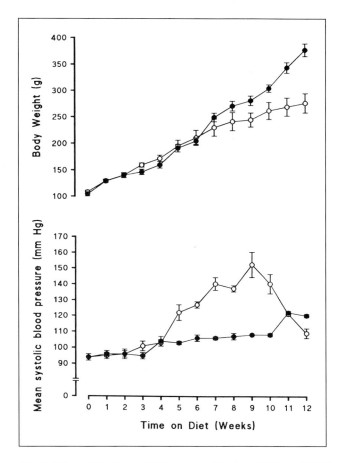

Fig. 1. Effect of feeding ad libitum a pyridoxine-deficient diet (○) or rat chow (●) on SBP and body weight in conscious rats. Blood pressure was measured by tail cuff plethysmography.

thyroxine replacement, blood pressure tended to normalize in the hypertensive hypothyroid patients. The mechanisms leading to hypertension in the hypothyroid condition are not known. However, in view of the relationship of hypothyroidism to vitamin B_6 deficiency which we have earlier shown [14, 15], we investigated the effect of vitamin B_6 deficiency in the adult male rat on blood pressure regulation.

Pyridoxine Deficiency: Animal Model of Hypertension

Male Sprague-Dawley rats (4–5 weeks of age, 95–110 g body weight) were randomly divided into 3 groups. One group was fed a pyridoxine-deficient diet and the second was pair-fed a pyridoxine-supplemented diet. The third group fed ad libitum a commercial rat chow for an equal length of time provided the normal controls. The systolic blood pressure (SBP) was measured indirectly once a week by tail cuff plethysmography in conscious animals [16] or directly from a cannula placed in the right carotid artery in anesthetized animals [17]. The SBP $\pm$ SE was 94 ± 2 mm Hg and the body weight $\pm$ SE was 108 ± 3 g at the start of the experiment. As shown in figure 1, the SBP increased to 103 ± 2 mm Hg in the 4th week on the deficient diet ($p < 0.01$) and to 122 ± 5 mm Hg in the 5th week, a rise of 20 mm Hg in 1 week ($p < 0.01$). The period between the 4th and 5th week on the deficient diet appears to be critical for the development of hypertension. There was a continued increase in SBP in subsequent weeks when it reached a peak value of about 140 mm Hg and began to fall starting in the 10th week on the pyridoxine-deficient diet. By the 12th week the values declined to normotensive (in some cases hypotensive) level, although they were still on the pyridoxine-deficient diet. The changes in systolic and diastolic pressures are given in table 1. Thus, the blood pressure changes in deficient rats can be divided into 3 phases: (1) prehypertensive (1–4 weeks); (2) hypertensive (5–11 weeks), and (3) posthyperten-

Table 1. Arterial blood pressure of vitamin-B_6-deficient and pyridoxine-supplemented (control) rats

Vitamin B_6 status	Arterial pressure, mm Hg	
	diastolic	systolic
Pyridoxine-supplemented (control)	77 ± 3	111 ± 2
Vitamin-V_6-deficient	105 ± 6*	147 ± 5**

Values are the means $\pm$ SEM of 5 separate determinations in each group. Control rats were supplemented with 50 mg pyridoxine/kg diet. * $p < 0.005$; ** $p < 0.001$; compared with control (Student's unpaired t test). (From Paulose et al. [17]; reprinted with permission of the publisher.)

sive (starting from the 12th week). The values for blood pressure obtained in the anesthetized rat [17] were comparable to those obtained in conscious rats by tail cuff plethysmography (fig. 1). The body weights of the rats on the 3 dietary treatments are also given in figure 1. It is significant to note that in the pair-fed controls on the pyridoxine-supplemented diet the SBP reached a value of 106 ± 2 mm Hg and remained at that level for the entire experimental period. Rats on ad libitum rat chow reached a body weight that was 100 g more than those on the other two diets. Their SBP started to increase around 10 weeks after the start of the experiment and reached a value of 120 mm Hg by the 12th week. This still was significantly lower than the SBP values for pyridoxine-deficient rats, during the hypertensive phase.

The rats on the deficient diet in these experiments were only moderately pyridoxine-deficient as judged by the decreases in serum and brain pyridoxal phosphate concentrations (table 2) and serum aminotransferase activities. They did not reveal any clinical signs of deficiency (fig. 2). Treatment with pyridoxine (10 mg/kg body weight) reversed the hypertension (table 3) in the deficient animals within 24 h [17].

Table 2. Effect of pyridoxine on pyridoxal 5′-phosphate, GABA, 5-HT, dopamine and norepinephrine levels in the hypothalamus of control and vitamin-B_6-deficient adult rats

Vitamin B_6 status	Pyridoxal 5′-phosphate nmol/g	GABA µmol/g	5-HT nmol/g	Dopamine nmol/g	Norepi-nephrine nmol/g
Group 1 Pyridoxine-supplemented (control)	3.49 ± 0.26	5.33 ± 0.16	1.38 ± 0.05	1.06 ± 0.20	3.34 ± 0.20
Group 2 Pyridoxine-treated control	3.26 ± 0.19	5.46 ± 0.21	1.49 ± 0.06	1.12 ± 0.16	3.29 ± 0.14
Group 3 Vitamin-B_6-deficient (experimental)	1.89 ± 0.16*	4.34 ± 0.16*	0.92 ± 0.04*	1.13 ± 0.18	3.03 ± 0.40
Group 4 Pyridoxine-treated experimental	3.06 ± 0.16	5.32 ± 0.21	1.85 ± 0.13**	1.21 ± 0.22	3.25 ± 0.28

Values are the means ± SEM of 10 separate determinations in each group. * $p < 0.01$: compared with groups 1, 2 and 4; ** $p < 0.01$: compared with groups 1, 2 and 3, respectively (Duncan's multiple-range test). (From Dakshinamurti and Paulose [18]; reprinted with permission of the publisher.)

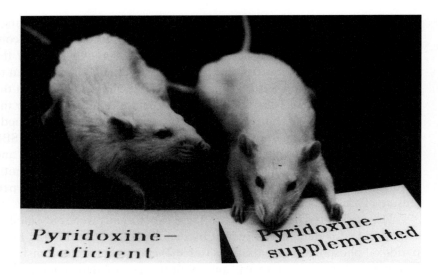

Fig. 2. Appearance of vitamin-B₆-deficient and control (pair-fed, pyridoxine-supplemented) rats at the 8th week.

Table 3. Effect of pyridoxine on pituitary thyrotropin (TSH) and serum thyroxine (T$_4$) triiodothyronine (T$_3$) and TSH in control and vitamin-B₆-deficient adult rats

Vitamin B₆ status	Pituitary TSH µg/mg protein	Serum TSH µg/l	Serum T$_4$ nmol/l	Serum T$_3$ nmol/l
Group 1 Pyridoxine-supplemented (control)	2.39 ± 0.18	3.91 ± 0.28	89 ± 5	0.98 ± 0.04
Group 2 Pyridoxine-treated control	2.43 ± 0.19	4.19 ± 0.82	92 ± 8	1.00 ± 0.06
Group 3 Vitamin-B₆-deficient (experimental)	5.90 ± 0.48*	1.94 ± 0.61*	64 ± 9*	0.84 ± 0.08*
Group 4 Pyridoxine-treated experimental	3.70 ± 0.27	3.46 ± 0.63	90 ± 3	1.15 ± 0.07

Values are the means ± SEM of 8–12 separate determinations in each group. * $p < 0.01$: compared with groups 1, 2 and 4, respectively (Duncan's multiple-range test). (From Dakshinamurti and Paulose [18]; reprinted with permission of the publisher.)

Characterization of Hypertension Induced by Vitamin B₆ Deficiency

The nature of the hypertension that developed in the pyridoxine-deficient animal needed to be characterized in an effort to identify the causative factor(s). Pyridoxine deficiency in rats could result in a hyperexcitable state. Seizures are seen in the pyridoxine-dependent state in humans as well as in experimental pyridoxine deficiency in young rats. Although spontaneous seizures were not observed in adult pyridoxine-deficient rats at this stage of deficiency, we investigated the effects of anticonvulsants such as phenytoin, valproic acid and diazepam on the blood pressure of these rats. A single dose of phenytoin (6 mg/100 g body weight i.p.) decreased the SBP in pyridoxine-deficient rats within 30 min from 135 ± 4 to 105 ± 3 mm Hg. The effect lasted for 6 h, at the end of which blood pressure was elevated again. Valproic acid (16 mg/100 g body weight i.p.) reversed the high SBP in the pyridoxine-deficient rats within 10 min from 133 ± 3 to 108 ± 2 mm Hg. The effect lasted for only 30 min. In similar short-term experiments, diazepam (8 mg/100 g body weight i.p.) had no effect on the systolic hypertension of pyridoxine-deficient rats. Both valproic acid, which is supposed to act through facilitation of inhibition [17], and phenytoin, which is supposed to act primarily on membranes [17], produce transient pharmacological effects. In contrast, pyridoxine administration resulted in a reversal of hypertension that lasted for several days after treatment, thus indicating the specificity of pyridoxine deficiency in the development of hypertension.

Role of Thyroid. A number of clinical studies have reported a correlation between hypothyroid condition and hypertension [12, 13]. Thyroxine administration not only corrected the hypothyroid condition but also normalized the blood pressure. In an earlier study from this laboratory it has been shown that vitamin B₆ deficiency in the rat causes hypothyroidism [14, 18, 19]. This hypothyroidism appears to originate from the hypothalamus [14]. Prior treatment with pyridoxine (10 mg/kg body weight) reversed the hypothyroidism and hypertension within 24 h [15, 19] (table 3). However, there was no indication that the hypothyroid condition initiated hypertension.

Sympathetic Nervous System. An association between hypertension and sympathetic stimulation has been observed in both hypertensive animals [20, 21] and humans [22]. Therefore, the possibility that the reversible hypertension seen in the deficient rat was related to sympathetic stimulation

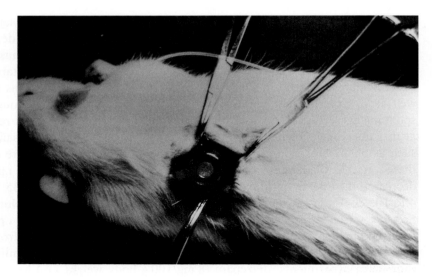

Fig. 3. Rat fitted with a vascular-access port. (From Paulose and Dakshinamurti [23], reprinted with permission of the publisher.)

Table 4. Effect of pyridoxine on plasma levels of norepinephrine and epinephrine in control and vitamin-B_6-deficient adult rats

Vitamin B_6 status	Norepinephrine nmol/l	Epinephrine nmol/l
Group 1 Pyridoxine-supplemented (control)	3.06 ± 0.28	1.89 ± 0.28
Group 2 Pyridoxine-treated control	3.44 ± 0.27	1.52 ± 0.16
Group 3 Vitamin-B_6-deficient (experimental)	$9.04 \pm 0.21*$	$4.39 \pm 0.21*$
Group 4 Pyridoxine-treated experimental	3.97 ± 0.32	2.73 ± 0.24

Values are the means ± SEM of 8–12 separate determinations in each group. Control rats were supplemented with 50 mg pyridoxine/kg diet. Pyridoxine treatment of control and vitamin-B_6-deficient rats involved a single intraperitoneal injection of 10 mg pyridoxine/10 kg body weight. * $p < 0.01$: compared with groups 1, 2 and 4, respectively (Duncan's multiple-range test). (From Paulose et al. [17]; reprinted with permission of the publisher.)

was considered. The concentration of norepinephrine in plasma is a valid reflection of sympathetic activity. However, blood samples have to be withdrawn from the conscious animal without trauma. Pyridoxine-deficient rats (in the hypertensive phase) and control rats (pyridoxine-supplemented) were implanted with vascular-access ports (Model SLA, Norfolk Medical Products, Skolie, Ill., USA) with catheterization of the jugular vein [23] (fig. 3). Within 24 h after surgery the rats returned to their preoperative blood pressure status. Blood samples were collected with least stress to the animals. Plasma catecholamines, after extraction using alumina, were assayed by a HPLC method with electrochemical detection [17, 23]. Both norepinephrine and epinephrine levels in the plasma of pyridoxine-deficient rats were nearly 3-fold higher ($p < 0.01$) compared with controls (table 4). Treatment of deficient rats with pyridoxine (10 mg/kg body weight) restored the blood pressure and catecholamine levels to normal within 24 h. Pyridoxine administration to the control rats had no significant effect on either of the indices measured. The complete reversibility of the hypertension in such a short time would preclude a permanent structural damage to the vessel wall of the deficient animal. The lesion might probably be at the level of neurotransmitter regulation. We also determined the norepinephrine turnover in the heart of the deficient as well as control groups by estimating the decrease in norepinephrine content [17] in the heart after inhibition of its synthesis with α-methyl-*p*-tyrosine [24]. No difference in myocardial norepinephrine content between two groups was seen (table 5). However, the norepinephrine turnover was significantly increased ($p < 0.05$) in the deficient rats compared to the controls, thus supporting the contention that peripheral sympathetic activity is increased in the pyridoxine-deficient animal.

Table 5. Myocardial norepinephrine (NE) content and turnover rates in pyridoxine-supplemented and pyridoxine-deficient adult rats

Animal status	NE content ng/g	NE turnover rate ng/g/h
Pyridoxine-supplemented	1,661.8 ± 241.8	30.0 ± 4.4
Pyridoxine-deficient	1,955.0 ± 260.8	106.6 ± 14.2*

Values represent the means ± SEM of 8 separate experiments. * $p < 0.05$. (From Viswanathan et al. [28]; reprinted with permission of the publisher.)

Pyridoxine and Central Neurotransmitter. Vitamin B_6 plays a crucial role in the functioning of the nervous system [19]. The putative neurotransmitters dopamine, norepinephrine, serotonin (5-HT), GABA and taurine as well as the polyamines are all synthesized by pyridoxal-phosphate-dependent enzymes. There is considerable variation in the affinities of various apoenzymes for pyridoxal phosphate. In view of this, during pyridoxine deficiency the pyridoxal-phosphate-dependent enzyme activities are decreased to varying extents, from no decrease to almost a complete depletion. As seen in table 2 [18], the contents of GABA and 5-HT in the deficient rat brain are significantly lower ($p < 0.01$) than those of control rats. Norepinephrine and dopamine contents were not affected in the hypertensive state of pyridoxine deficiency. This is crucial for understanding the role of each neurotransmitter in the hypertension induced by pyridoxine deficiency.

Role of Central Norepinephrine. The effects of antihypertensive drugs such as clonidine and α-methyldopa were tested in pyridoxine-deficient rats fitted with vascular-access ports. Basal SBP of the deficient rats recorded by tail cuff plethysmography was stable. Following this, the drug was administered through the port twice daily at 9.00 and 17.00 h for 4 days. One group of deficient rats received clonidine (10 µg/kg body weight), while a second group received α-methyldopa (40 mg/kg body weight) and the third group of rats the vehicle (saline) through the port for the same time period. Blood pressure was monitored on the 5th day of experiment. Both drugs reduced the SBP of deficient rats to the normal level (table 6). Clonidine-like drugs exert their cardiovascular-depressive effects mainly through a centrally mediated sympathetic inhibition due to a stimulation of α₂-adrenoceptors [25].

In view of the hypotensive effect of the α₂-receptor agonists, the possibility of decreased adrenergic output to the brainstem was examined. The kinetics of ligand binding to α₂-adrenoceptors were examined using the ligand [³H]-*p*-aminoclonidine binding to crude synaptosomal membrane preparations from the brainstem of pyridoxine-deficient and control rats [26]. Scatchard analysis of the specific binding data [27] shown in table 7 indicates a significant increase in the B_{max} of the high- and low-affinity [³H]-*p*-aminoclonidine binding to α₂-adrenoceptors in the brainstem of deficient rats compared to controls, without any change in the binding affinity. This would indicate a chronic underexposure of these receptors to endogenous norepinephrine. Such an assumption is supported by a de-

Table 6. Effect of clonidine and α-methyldopa on SBP of pyridoxine-deficient adult rats

Group	SBP, mm Hg
Pyridoxine-deficient	134 ± 4*
Pyridoxine-deficient + clonidine (10 µg/kg)	107 ± 3
Pyridoxine-deficient + α-methyldopa (40 µg/kg)	105 ± 4

Values are the means ± SEM of 5 separate determinations. * $p < 0.01$: compared with groups 2 and 3. (From Viswanathan et al. [28]; reprinted with permission of the publisher.)

Table 7. p-[3,5-^{3}H]-aminoclonidine binding to the α-adrenoceptors in the brainstem of control and pyridoxine-deficient adult rats

Group	High-affinity receptors		Low-affinity receptors	
	B_{max} fmol/mg protein	K_d nM	B_{max} fmol/mg protein	K_d nM
Control	51 ± 3	1.65 ± 0.33	172 ± 16	7.48 ± 1.41
Pyridoxine-deficient	89 ± 9*	1.96 ± 0.54	247 ± 9*	9.17 ± 0.47

Values are the means ± SEM of separate experiments. * $p < 0.01$: compared with control group. (From Viswanathan et al. [28]; reprinted with permission of the publisher.)

crease ($p < 0.05$) in the norepinephrine metabolite 3-methoxy-4-hydroxy-phenylglycol levels in the brainstem of deficient rats [28], indicating a low turnover of norepinephrine in the brainstem. This was in contrast to norepinephrine turnover in the heart (table 5). The central mechanism for maintaining normal blood pressure is regulated by the balance between sympathetic and parasympathetic nervous system tonicities in the brainstem [29, 30]. The antihypertensive effect of clonidine-like drugs is due to their agonistic activity at central α$_2$-adrenoreceptors in the nucleus tractus solitarii. When these receptors in the nucleus tractus solitarii are stimulated, inhibitory neurons of the vasomotor center are activated. This reduces the sympathetic outflow (which originates from the vasomotor center) to the peripheral vasculature, heart and kidney. As a result, peripheral vascular tone, heart rate and renin release are decreased, resulting in a reduction in total peripheral resistance and cardiovascular output [31]. It has been suggested that the regulation of central adrenergic receptors is not confined to adrenergic mechanisms alone but requires a serotonergic component [31]. As seen in the down-regulation of β-adrenergic receptors induced by antidepressant drugs [32], modification of α_2-adrenergic receptors could require a degree of serotonergic input. Lesioning of the central serotonergic pathways using 5,7-dihydroxytryptamine led to an increase in the B_{max} of [^{3}H]-p-aminoclonidine binding. In the pyridoxine-deficient rat there is a significant reduction in the 5-HT content of the brainstem [18].

Role of Serotonin and γ-Aminobutyric Acid. The decrease in 5-HT in brain regions of the pyridoxine-deficient rat (table 2) has physiological relevance to the central regulation of blood pressure. This decrease is the synaptic release of 5-HT in the deficient rat brain, as indicated by the increase in postsynaptic receptor density [27].

5-HT, when administered into the brain, elicits complex cardiovascular responses. Depressor, pressor or biphasic responses were reported [33–35]. This reflects the nonhomogeneous nature of brain 5-HT neurons which subserve different functions [36]. The receptors that mediate various cardiovascular effects of 5-HT are different. The development of specific agonists and antagonists that exert activity at different 5-HT receptors has contributed to our understanding of the role of 5-HT in physiopathological conditions [37]. Substances that have agonistic activity at the 5-HT$_1$-like receptors [38, 39] may mediate vasodilator effects, while the 5-HT$_2$ receptor agonists cause vasoconstriction [40, 41]. The initial short-lasting hypotension due to reflex bradycardia (von Bezold-Jarisch reflex) is mediated by 5-HT$_3$ receptors. 5-HT$_1$-like receptors [42] have been shown to be heterogeneous and subdivided into 4 subclasses. Specific agonists and antagonists have been developed for 5-HT$_{1A}$- and 5-HT$_{1B}$-like receptors [42]. 5-HT$_{1A}$ agonists like 8-hydroxy-2-(di-n-propylamino)-Tetralin (8-OH-DPAT), flesinoxan [43], reduce blood pressure and have attracted much clinical interest. A large body of evidence indicates that serotonergic neurons participate in the regulation of sympathetic nervous activity and, therefore, of blood pressure [31, 44]. As noted earlier, modification of α_2-adrenoceptors could require a degree of serotonergic input. 5-HT$_{1A}$ agonists have been shown to reduce blood pressure and sympathetic nerve activity [45, 46], indicating that the serotonergic receptors involved in the

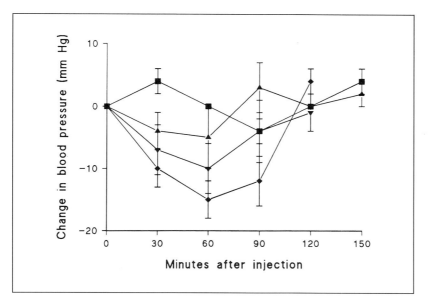

Fig. 4. Effect of intravenous injection of various doses of the 5-HT$_{1A}$ agonist, 8-OH-DPAT, in anesthetized pyridoxine-deficient hypertensive rats. ■ = Saline; ▲ = 10 µg 8-OH-DPAT/kg; ▼ = 100 µg 8-OH-DPAT/kg; ♦ = 1,000 µg 8-OH-DPAT/kg.

regulation of α_2-adrenoceptors are 5-HT$_{1A}$-like. It is probable, therefore, that the decrease in serotonergic activity of the brainstem of pyridoxine-deficient rats is responsible for the alteration in α_2-adrenergic function and the resultant sympathetic stimulation. This possibility was tested in acute experiments.

After deficient rats were anesthetized with pentobarbitone, the right carotid artery was cannulated and connected to a pressure transducer and a chart recorder. Injections were made through a cannula in the left jugular vein. Injection of 8-OH-DPAT (10–100 µg/kg body weight) reduced the mean blood pressure ($p < 0.01$). A 10-µg/kg dose caused a reduction of 30 mm Hg. Although recovery was seen after 90 min, the blood pressure returned to the preinjection level after 150 min. A 100-µg/kg dose reduced the SBP to the same extent as the 10-µg/kg dose, but the antihypertensive effect lasted for several hours. A 1-µg/kg dose did not consistently affect the blood pressure in all the rats studied (fig. 4). A comparison of our results with other reports of its use in spontaneously hypertensive rats

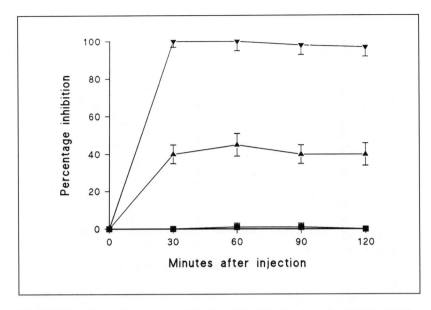

Fig. 5. Effect of prior intravenous injection (15 min) of various doses of the 5-HT$_{1A}$ antagonist, spiroxatrine, on 8-OH-DPAT (40 nmol/kg)-induced hypotension in anesthetized pyridoxine-deficient hypertensive rat. Spiroxatrine was administered at 40 nmol/kg (■), 60 nmol/kg (▲) and 80 nmol/kg (▼).

(SHR) [45] indicated that the pyridoxine-deficient rats are more sensitive to the antihypertensive effect of 8-OH-DPAT.

In order to examine whether the 5-HT$_{1A}$ receptor mediates the antihypertensive activity of 8-OH-DPAT, spiroxatrine, a specific 5-HT$_{1A}$ antagonist, was injected 15 min before 8-OH-DPAT. Spiroxatrine, at a dose of 50 nmol/kg, inhibited nearly 50% of the antihypertensive effect of 40 nmol/kg (10 µg/kg), but at 80 nmol/kg totally abolished the antihypertensive effect of the agonist (fig. 5). These results suggest that pyridoxine-deficient (hypertensive) rats are very sensitive to 5-HT$_{1A}$ agonists, and this could be because of underexposure of these receptors to 5-HT, due to its decreased synthesis.

In order to test this assumption, we studied the kinetics of the binding of [^{3}H]-8-OH-DPAT to membrane preparations from brain regions. Preliminary data from a Scatchard analysis of specific binding of the ligand to membrane preparations from cerebral cortex of moderately pyridoxine-deficient rats indicate an increase in sensitivity of 5-HT$_{1A}$ receptors with no change in the sensitivity of 5-HT$_2$ receptors. This is in keeping with the sensitivity to the hypotensive effect of 5-HT$_{1A}$ agonists exhibited by the pyridoxine-deficient hypertensive rat. Further investigation would indicate if there is a profile of varying changes in the sensitivity of the different 5-HT receptors in various brain regions.

In the experiments reported above, sympathetic nervous activity or any parameter that reflects this activity was not monitored, but our results are consistent with the concept that the agonistic activity at this receptor site caused inhibition of sympathetic nervous activity, resulting in reduction in SBP. Injection of pyridoxine (10 mg/kg body weight) not only reduces SBP and sympathetic activity, but also restored 5-HT and GABA levels to control values [18].

Central GABAergic neurons have been suggested to cause hypotensive effects. Administration of GABA or its agonists such as muscimol into brain causes a reduction in blood pressure [47–49], an effect blocked by its antagonist bicuculline [50]. A reduced sympathetic outflow has been suggested in the mediation of the cardiovascular effects of GABA [51]. Pharmacological and binding studies are needed to assess the role of GABA in this model of hypertension.

Peripheral Effects of Pyridoxine Deficiency. Disturbances in calcium regulation have been suggested to be the cause of hypotension (see section on vitamin D). Increased peripheral resistance resulting from increased permeability of vascular smooth muscle plasma membrane to Ca^{2+} is thought to be one of the mechanisms of hypertension. In the SHR model of hypertension, a number of studies have demonstrated increasing resting calcium influx in the vascular smooth muscle [52–55]. Isometric tension development and calcium uptake in caudal artery segments from pyridoxine-deficient and control rats were examined [56]. Isometric tension development in the caudal artery was studied in small arterial rings which were placed in a 10-ml capacity organ bath containing oxygenated Krebs-Henseleit medium (pH 7.4, 37 °C, aerated with 95% O_2 + 5% CO_2). Arterial rings were suspended on steel wire loops and attached to a mechanical force transducer (Grass FT03). Signals were amplified and recorded on a Gould 260, 6-channel chart recorder.

A significantly greater decrease in resting, spontaneous tone of caudal artery segments was observed when EGTA was added to the bathing medium of the arterial rings obtained from pyridoxine-deficient rats (fig. 6). The decrease in unstimulated isometric tension observed in response to 5 mM EGTA-Na was 0.25 ± 0.03 mN per milligram of control arterial tissue compared with 0.72 ± 0.72 mN in arterial tissue from pyridoxine-deficient rats. The active tension response to depolarization with 50 mM potassium was not different between control and deficient artery segments. Similar to the EGTA effect, addition of nifedipine also induced a decrease in tone in arterial segments from pyridoxine-deficient rats but not in control rats. Spontaneous rhythmic contractions were much larger and more frequent in artery segments from deficient rats. These could also be eliminated by nifedipine. Recovery of tone in arterial segments was noticed when Ca^{2+} was added back to the medium. The α-adrenergic blocker and vasodilator, phenoxybenzamine (1 μM), did not alter the tone in any of the arterial segments in vitro.

Calcium uptake was studied in caudal artery segments (10 mm long) of pyridoxine-deficient and control rats. They were equilibrated for 60 min in Krebs-Henseleit medium, oxygenated and maintained at 37 °C. The segments were then incubated for various times in Krebs-Henseleit medium containing 5 μCi/ml ^{45}Ca. At the end of the incubation period the segments were plunged into ice-cold lanthanum solution of the following composition (in mM): NaCl 122; KCl 5.9; $MgCl_2$ 1.25; $LaCl_3$ 50; glucose 11, and Tris-maleate (pH 6.8) 15. After 30 min in lanthanum solution the artery segments were blotted and weighed. The segments were then digested in 100 μl of concentrated perchloric acid/nitric acid (1:1 v/v) for 18 h, scintillant added and the radioactivity determined. The dpm were converted to apparent content of ^{45}Ca according to the formula: ^{45}Ca content (mmol/kg weight) = (dpm in tissue/wet weight in kg)×(mmol Ca per liter of medium/dpm per liter of medium).

Calcium uptake was significantly increased in the caudal artery of pyridoxine-deficient rats (fig. 6). Nifedipine exerted a dose-dependent inhibition on the uptake of ^{45}Ca into the caudal artery of pyridoxine-deficient rats (fig. 6). Our results demonstrate that there is increased calcium influx into the caudal artery of pyridoxine-deficient rats that is mediated through calcium channels, since calcium channel blockers as well as lowering of extracellular calcium corrected the defect. A similar increased uptake of ^{45}Ca into the aortae of SHR compared to those from normotensive Wistar-Kyoto (WKY) rats has been reported [54]. The results presented here on artery segments from pyridoxine-deficient rats using EGTA and calcium replenishment suggest that smooth muscle membranes from the caudal artery of deficient rats leak calcium similar to that reported for

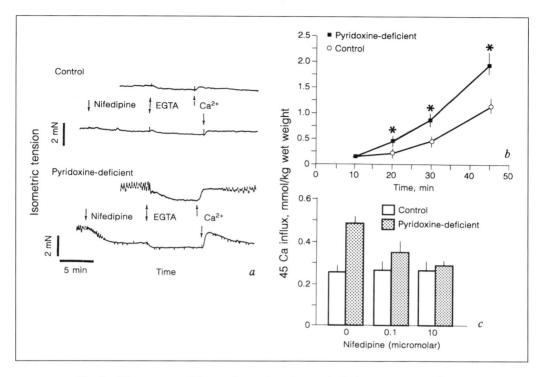

Fig. 6. a Time course of isometric tension changes in isolated segments of caudal artery from control (top two traces) and pyridoxine-deficient rats (bottom two traces). The effect of addition of 1 µM nifedipine or/and 5 mM EGTA-Na or 2.5 mM calcium is shown, as indicated by the arrows. *b* Cold-lanthanum-resistant calcium uptake into caudal artery strips is shown here as a function of time. ■ = Uptake in strips from pyridoxine-deficient animals; ○ = same from control animals. Bars represent SEM for each time point in each group. * p < 0.05. *c* Effect of nifedipine on lanthanum-resistant calcium influx into caudal arteries from pyridoxine-deficient and control rats after 30 min of incubation. Data from 8 rats with SE bars are shown. (From Viswanathan et al. [56]; reproduced with permission of the publisher.)

the aorta of SHR [57]. Our results indicate a greater leakiness to calcium which results in elevated cytosolic calcium and, thus, an increase in the tone of blood vessels. This would contribute significantly to the increase in blood pressure observed in pyridoxine-deficient animals.

A number of investigations in hypertensive and normotensive animals and humans suggest that increased dietary calcium intake lowers blood

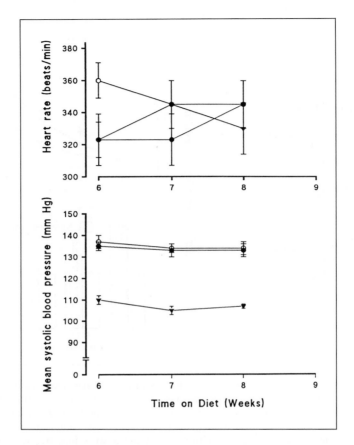

Fig. 7. Effect of varying dietary levels of calcium on the development of hypertension induced by pyridoxine deficiency. The rats were randomly divided into 3 groups and assigned to a pyridoxine-deficient diet containing, respectively 0.5% (○), 1% (●) or 1.5% (▼) calcium. Blood pressure was measured by tail cuff plethysmography in conscious animals. Each value represents the mean ± SE of 8 rats.

pressure [58–61], while low dietary calcium [62] enhances the development of hypertension. We examined this possibility in pyridoxine-deficient rats.

In one experiment, pyridoxine-deficient diets containing, respectively, 0.5, 1 and 1.5% calcium were prepared. Rats were fed one of the above pyridoxine-deficient diets and blood pressure was recorded by tail cuff

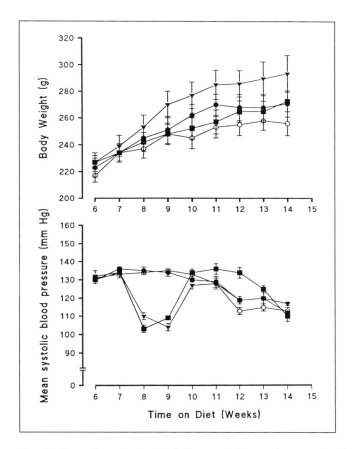

Fig. 8. Effect of varying levels of dietary calcium on hypertension induced by pyridoxine deficiency. All rats were fed the standard pyridoxine-deficient (0.5 % calcium) diet ad libitum for 6 weeks and after development of hypertension were divided into 4 groups. They were then placed on a pyridoxine-deficient diet containing, respectively, 0.5 % (○), 1 % (●), 1.5 % (▼) or 2.5 % (■) calcium. After measuring blood pressure in the 9th week all the groups were again changed to the standard pyridoxine-deficient diet. Blood pressure was measured by tail cuff plethysmography in conscious animals. Each value represents the mean ± SE of 8 rats.

plethysmography every week. As shown in figure 7, only rats placed on pyridoxine-deficient diets containing 0.5 and 1 % calcium developed hypertension, while rats fed the higher (1.5%) calcium-containing pyridoxine-deficient diet failed to develop hypertension. Thus, the development of hypertension by vitamin B_6 deprivation is inhibited by higher dietary calcium content.

In another experiment, rats were placed on the pyridoxine-deficient diet (containing 0.5% calcium). Blood pressure was monitored by tail cuff plethysmography every week. After 5 weeks when hypertension developed in the rats, they were divided randomly into 4 groups and placed on one of the pyridoxine-deficient diets containing, respectively, 0.5, 1, 1.5 and 2.5% calcium. Rats on the 0.5 and 1% calcium diet continued to be hypertensive, but those on 1.5% and 2.5% calcium became normotensive (fig. 8). Thus, as in other hypertensive animal models, dietary calcium supplementation does inhibit the expression of hypertension in the moderately pyridoxine-deficient rat.

The moderately pyridoxine-deficient adult rat is another animal model for essential hypertension in humans. Although the hypertension is not as severe as in the SHR, it shares with SHR features like the associated sympathetic stimulation and smooth muscle leakiness to calcium. The advantage of this animal model is the response to pyridoxine treatment which is complete and takes place within 24 h.

Vitamin D

Vitamin D acting in association with parathyroid hormone (PTH) has a pivotal role in calcium homeostasis. PTH is the primary regulator of renal handling of calcium. Skeletal mobilization of calcium requires both PTH and 1,25-dihydroxycholecalciferol [1,25$(OH)_2D_3$], the active metabolite of cholecalciferol (vitamin D_3). This active form of vitamin D is formed in the kidney by the action of the 1-hydroxylase on 25-hydroxycholecalciferol, a metabolite of vitamin D_3, formed in the liver. The kidney hydroxylase is regulated by PTH. 1,25$(OH)_2D_3$ is active in increasing the intestinal absorption of calcium as well as phosphorus. There is also evidence to indicate that 1,25$(OH)_2D_3$ may also directly suppress the secretion of PTH [63]. In view of the regulation of PTH secretion by serum calcium, the interacting homeostatic cycle among PTH, the active form of vitamin D_3 and serum calcium is complete.

The early report [64] of the negative correlation between hardness of water and prevalence of cardiovascular disease was indicated to be related to the calcium content of the hard water [65]. McCarron et al. [66] and

Harlan et al. [67] have analyzed the data collected between 1971 and 1975 by the US Health and Nutrition Examination Survey I with a sampling of 20,000 Americans. They concluded that the reduced intake of calcium was the primary nutritional marker of hypertension and that the increase in SBP correlated strongly with the decrease in dietary calcium intake. Potassium intake was also lower in hypertensives than in normotensives. Several reports of the beneficial effects of calcium supplementation on hypertension in humans [68, 69] support the suggestion of a deficient calcium intake. At least 23 subsequent publications have verified the finding of an inverse relationship between dietary calcium intake and blood pressure [70]. The report of Witteman et al. [71] extends these correlations to females as well. Thus, the inverse correlation between calcium intake and blood pressure seems to apply to all age, gender, racial and socioeconomic groups.

A large number of studies in hypertensive humans and animals have explored the relationships among vitamin D metabolites, serum PTH and serum calcium. Early clinical observations [72] indicated an enhanced function of the parathyroids in essential hypertension. This was followed by reports of lowered serum ionized calcium concentration in hypertensive humans [73]. The potential application of this concept of aberrant Ca^{2+}-vitamin D_3-PTH axis in understanding the pathophysiology of essential hypertension and providing appropriate therapy has resulted in extensive clinical investigations as well as in experimental work with various animal models of essential hypertension. There have been contradictory reports in this emerging area of investigation [74].

McCarron [75] has suggested that calcium may be more important than sodium in the pathogenesis of essential hypertension. A decreased intake of calcium or its increased excretion in urine could lead to decreased serum ionized calcium concentration. Hypercalciuria has been shown in animal models of hypertension as well as in human hypertensives [59, 76]. This could be due to a renal calcium leak [75].

Schedl et al. [77] have reported that serum ionized calcium levels were lower and serum immunoreactive PTH levels higher in SHR than in WKY controls. Total serum calcium levels were the same in both patients with essential hypertension and their normotensive controls [73]. This is true also of SHR and their WKY control rats [16]. Schedl et al. [77] also noted that the concentration of $1,25(OH)_2D_3$ in the serum of SHR was normal although it was low in relation to the high level of serum PTH in these rats. Intestinal absorption of calcium has been shown to be decreased in SHR, suggesting unresponsiveness of the gastrointestinal tract to the active vitamin D metabolite [77–80]. Lucas et al. [80] have reported a reduction in circulating $1,25(OH)_2D_3$ in 12- to 14-week-old male SHR, results at variance with those of Schedl et al. [77]. The contradictory observations could be ascribed to differences in experimental conditions including the levels of calcium, vitamin D and phosphorus in the diets used. Young et al. [81] have examined the plasma levels of $1,25(OH)_2D_3$ in SHR and WKY rats in response to several known stimuli such as infusion of PTH or cyclic AMP in thyroparathyroidectomized rats as well as dietary phosphorus depletion. Under all these conditions the response in SHR was submaximal when compared with WKY controls. They suggested a decreased 1-hydroxylase activity or an enhanced metabolic clearance of the active form of vitamin D as contributing to the low plasma $1,25(OH)_2D_3$ levels observed. Hsu et al. [82] reported that renal clearance studies failed to show a defect in renal calcium handling in the SHR. The decrease in net intestinal calcium flux in these rats was corrected by administration of vitamin D. They also showed that the mobilization of calcium after PTH infusion was not different between SHR and WKY controls. Thus, an impairment of vitamin D metabolism possibly at the level of the kidney 1-hydroxylase has also been suggested by them to be the primary defect in SHR. In addition, the unresponsiveness of the gastrointestinal tract of the hypertensive rat to the active form of vitamin D has also been indicated to contribute to the impairment of calcium homeostasis. The observation that the total serum calcium is unaltered between normo- and hypertensive humans and animals will argue against this possibility.

Results of clinical studies show a similar pattern. A decrease in serum ionized calcium has been reported in hypertensives [73], particularly those who are salt-sensitive and have low renin [83]. As against the decrease in serum ionized calcium, intracellular calcium concentration is increased in platelets, lymphocytes and proximal tubular cells of hypertensives [70], as well as in cell lines derived from hypertensive animals and humans. Cellular calcium handling defects could represent multiple disturbances in different cell lines or might reflect the effect of a single, primary defect in the regulation of the calcium pump, in the binding of calcium to intracellular binding proteins or in the response to local circulating factors that activate calmodulin. As a result of a genetic defect or an inadequate intake of calcium, a disorder of cellular calcium transport develops that leads to decrease in intestinal absorption and impaired reabsorption of calcium. If hypertension results from an inherent abnormality in calcium homeostasis, would increased dietary intake overcome this disorder? McCarron [70] noted that increased dietary calcium lowered blood pressure in at least 3 normotensive rat strains as well as in nongenetic models of hypertension, and contended that increased calcium intake might modify systemic factors such as the calcium-regulating hormones which, in turn, modify the expression of the genetic defect. The reversion of this defect might reflect a change in the regulation of the Mg^{2+}/Ca^{2+}-ATPase which results from increased exposure of the cell to calcium as the calcium pump is regulated by both Ca^{2+} and calmodulin.

Resnick [83] has attempted to reconcile the seemingly contradictory situation of a direct relationship between blood pressure and cytosolic free calcium, serum total calcium, increased urinary excretion of calcium, the direct peripheral and renal vasoconstrictor action of calcium ion and the hypertension of hypercalcemic states with the widespread finding that oral calcium supplementation can lower blood pressure in human hypertensive and normotensive populations. Calcium metabolism seems to be altered in hypertension in both directions away from normal values. Serum ionized calcium levels are decreased in low-renin hypertensives. The opposite is the case in high-renin hypertensives [83]. Such a diversity among hypertensives in regard to calcium metabolism is seen if they are categorized according to the sensitivity of their blood pressure to intake of sodium chloride. These criteria which are useful to determine the efficacy of oral calcium treatment of hypertensives suggest a relationship among renin, sodium and calcium in the pathogenesis of hypertension.

A more direct role for vitamin D in regulating blood pressure is suggested by other observations. In the deoxycorticosterone acetate salt model of hypertension, dietary manipulation of vitamin D has been shown to result in alterations of blood pressure without change in serum calcium level [84, 85], indicating a direct effect on blood pressure regulation. In line with this contention are observations of a decrease in the integral membrane calcium-binding proteins in the SHR [86]. This protein is regulated by vitamin D. Vascular tissue contains receptors for both the calcium-regulating hormones, PTH and $1,25(OH)_2D_3$. As the circulating levels of these hormones are regulated by dietary calcium, they are potential mediators of the effects of dietary calcium [85]. The incubation of isolated vascular smooth muscle cells with either PTH or $1,25(OH)_2D_3$ stimulates $^{45}Ca^{2+}$ uptake [87]. Short-term incubation of intact mesenteric resistance vessels with either $1,25(OH)_2D_3$ or PTH significantly modified calcium transport evoked by exposure to norepinephrine. $1,25(OH)_2D_3$ dampened the calcium transport in vessels from normotensive rats, whereas it increased the transport in vessels isolated from SHR. PTH reduced the calcium transport in the normotensive WKY and had minimal effect on calcium transport in the SHR [70]. These results suggest a direct intracellular effect of the calcium-regulating hormones on calcium release and storage by intact resistance vessels. The mechanism of action of these hormones in regulating cellular calcium uptake or transport in resistance vessels is not known.

In another work, MacCarthy et al. [88] have examined the effect of the active form of vitamin D on growth of cultured vascular smooth muscle cells and found it to suppress its growth. $1,25(OH)_2D_3$ antagonizes the mitogenic effect of epidermal growth factor on proliferation of vascular smooth muscle cells. This effect is not mediated through alteration of the binding of epidermal growth factor to vascular smooth muscle cells.

In a series of clinical trials, Lind et al. [89, 90] have examined the hypotensive potential of vitamin D. In a double-blind, placebo-controlled study they found that blood pressure was lowered by vitamin D during long-term treatment of patients with intermittent hypercalcemia. The mechanism of this action is not known although there are possible explanations. The increased calcium load due to increased intestinal calcium absorption mediated by vitamin D might cause natriuresis and, thus, lower blood pressure through a diuretic action [89]. Inhibition by calcium of calcium transport through calcium channel blockade has been demonstrated experimentally [91]. In a further study of this effect of active vitamin D on hypercalcemic patients, Lind et al. [92] found that both serum total and ionized calcium levels were increased. At the same time there was a significant reduction of diastolic blood pressure. The hypotensive effect of vitamin D was inversely related to the pretreatment serum levels of $1,25(OH)_2D_3$ and additive to antihypertensive medications.

In summary, epidemiological, clinical and experimental investigations all indicate a relationship between the plasma levels of $1,25(OH)_2D_3$ and hypertension. This includes the vitamin-D-mediated significant reduction in blood pressure of hypertensives. The mechanism of the action of vitamin D in this is not understood yet. Both a direct effect, acting on cell membranes, and an indirect effect, acting through enhancement of calcium transport, are indicated.

Vitamin E

It is well established that unsaturated fatty acid hydroperoxidation causes damage to cell membranes and tissue components in a variety of pathological conditions, including preeclampsia of pregnancy [93–95]. Free-radical-mediated peroxidation of membrane polyunsaturated fatty acids results in alteration of membrane integrity and its function [96, 97]. The products of free radical oxidation have powerful effects on processes such as platelet aggregation [98–100] and smooth muscle stimulation. Vitamin E is an endogenous antioxidant breaking the chain of lipid peroxidation in cell membranes and preventing the formation of lipid hydroperoxides [101, 102]. It also stabilizes the membrane probably by acting as a filler in the phospholipid bilayer [103], an effect unrelated to its function as an antioxidant [104, 105]. Also its ability to regulate cell turnover rate may also contribute to its protective role [106]. Vitamin E is an integral part of the antioxidant defence mechanisms [107].

An increase in peripheral resistance in the small blood vessels due to atherosclerosis, fibrosis or damage to the vessel wall is believed to be an important contributor to the development of hypertension [108]. Increased lipid hydroperoxides derived from polyunsaturated fatty acids by the action of free radicals have been shown to cause damage to endothelial cells of the blood vessels [2, 109, 110]. Damage to the endothelium of porcine pulmonary artery caused by lipid peroxides [111] can be prevented by vitamin E [112]. Injection of lipid peroxides to rabbits causes marked denudation of endothelial cells of the aorta [113]. Plasma lipid peroxide levels and the susceptibility of blood cells to peroxidation are significantly increased in hypertensive patients [114]. Thus, vascular lesions seen in essential hypertension could be produced by free radicals [115]. Furthermore, lipid peroxides also reduce the vasodilator prostacyclin production by a direct effect [116] as well as by depleting precursor polyunsaturated fatty acids [108, 117, 118]. Lack of prostacyclin results in platelet aggregation. Endothelial damage reduces the ability of vasodilators like acetylcholine to relax vascular smooth muscle [119].

Tissue vitamin E levels were significantly lower in SHR than in normotensive WKY controls [120]. Even when vitamin-E-depleted SHR and WKY controls were given identical doses of vitamin E orally the levels of vitamin E in the plasma and liver of SHR were significantly lower than in controls, suggesting the possibility of a defect in the absorption of vitamin E in SHR. Available literature data are inadequate to determine whether there is a cause-effect relationship between vitamin E status and hypertension in 12- to 15-week-old SHR. It would be of interest to examine if this absorptive defect precedes the expression of hypertension in the SHR.

Vitamin-E-deficient rats develop vascular pathologies similar to those seen in hypertensive human preeclampsia [121, 122]. However, vitamin E deprivation did not alter blood pressure. Hubel et al. [119] studied the effect of long-term lipid peroxidative stress produced by dietary deprivation of vitamin E on vascular function. A functional vitamin-E-deficient state was indicated in these rats by the increase in tissue thiobarbituric-acid-reactive material and by increase in spontaneous hemolysis of washed red cells in female rats fed the vitamin-E-deficient diet for 22 weeks. SBP was not altered [121]. However, there was increased pressor responsiveness to angiotensin II and decreased relaxation response to acetylcholine in the mesenteric artery of the deficient rats. These changes are generally associated with the hypertensive state [123–126]. Hubel et al. [119] concluded that vitamin E deficiency in the rat produces marked changes in vascular function associated with lipid peroxidation and endothelial cell structure abnormalities. Although a hypertensive state has not been shown to result from vitamin E deprivation in rats, an increased responsiveness to hypertensive stimuli has been demonstrated in the vitamin-E-deficient rat.

Conclusions

Among the vitamins, pyridoxine (vitamin B_6) and cholecalciferol (vitamin D) seem to have significant influences on blood pressure regulation. The effect of vitamin E seems to be indirect, based on the maintenance of the integrity of membranes. The case for vitamin B_6 as a regulator of arterial blood pressure is strong. Acting through central serotonergic and GABAergic neurotransmission, sympathetic stimulation is affected under conditions of excess or deficiency. In addition, there is a peripheral effect on resistance vessels mediated by changes in calcium transport. It is possible that both central and peripheral actions might be mediated by a common mechanism acting through calcium transport. The fact that higher levels of dietary calcium supplementation to pyridoxine-deficient hypertensive rats result in lowering of SBP would argue in favor of such a common mechanism. As hypertension develops only during moderate deficiency of pyridoxine, it raises the question whether some hypertensives could have a moderate deficiency of pyridoxine or a defect in the conversion of pyridoxine to pyridoxal phosphate. Assessment of the pyridoxine vitamin status of borderline hypertensives might yield valuable information.

Vitamin D is directly involved in regulation of calcium homeostasis. Conditions associated with a deficiency of vitamin D or its conversion to the active form, $1,25(OH)_2D_3$, would have profound effect on intestinal calcium absorption and, thus, indirectly on regulation of blood pressure. A more direct effect mediated through the synthesis of calcium-binding proteins or through a modificaiton of calcium transport evoked by norepinephrine is also indicated. Although the mechanisms of action of these effects are not understood yet, clinical trials point to a hypotensive potential of vitamin D.

References

1   Cleary RE, Lumeng L, Li T-K: Maternal and fetal plasma levels of pyridoxal phosphate at term: Adequacy of vitamin B_6 supplementation during pregnancy. Am J Obstet Gynecol 1975;121:25–28.
2   Brophy MH, Siiteri PK: Pyridoxal phosphate and hypertensive disorders of pregnancy. Am J Obstet Gynecol 1975;121:1075–1079.
3   Klieger JA, Altshuller CH, Krakow G, et al: Abnormal pyridoxine metabolism in toxemia of pregnancy. Ann NY Acad Sci 1969;166:288–296.
4   Hunt IF, Murphy NJ, Clever AE, et al: Zinc supplementation during pregnancy: Effects on selected blood constituents and on progress and outcome of pregnancy in low-income women of Mexican desert. Am J Clin Nutr 1984;40:508–521.
5   Flowers CE Jr: Magnesium sulfate in obstetrics. Am J Obstet Gynecol 1965;91: 763–772.
6   Pritchard JA: The use of magnesium ion in the management of eclamptogenic toxemias. Surg Gynecol Obstet 1955;100:131–140.
7   Brophy MH: Zinc preeclampsia and γ-aminobutyric acid. J Obstet Gynecol 1990; 163:242–243.
8   Potter LF, Beevers DG: The possible mechanisms of alcohol associated hypertension. Ann Intern Med 1983;98:97–102.
9   Fuller JH: Epidemiology of hypertension associated with diabetes mellitus. Hypertension 1985;7(suppl II):3–7.
10 Lumeng L, Li T-K: Vitamin B_6 metabolism in chronic alcohol abuse: Pyridoxal phosphate levels in plasma and the effects of acetaldehyde on pyridoxal phosphate synthesis and degradation in human erythrocytes. J Clin Invest 1974;53:693–704.
11 Davis RE, Calder JS, Curnow DH: Serum pyridoxal and folate concentration in diabetes. Pathology 1976;8:151–156.
12 Bing RF, Briggs RSJ, Burden AC, et al: Reversible hypertension and hypothyroidism. Clin Endocrinol 1980;13:339–342.

13 Saito I, Ito K, Saruta T: Hypothyroidism as a cause of hypertension. Hypertension 1983;5:112–115.

14 Dakshinamurti K, Paulose CS, Thliveris JA, et al: Thyroid function in pyridoxine-deficient young rats. J Endocrinol 1985;104:339–344.

15 Dakshinamurti K, Paulose CS, Vriend J: Hypothyroidism of hypothalamic origin in pyridoxine-deficient rats. J Endocrinol 1986;109:345–349.

16 Bunang RD, Butterfield J: Tail cuff blood pressure measurement without external preheating in awake rats. Hypertension 1982;4:898–903.

17 Paulose CS, Dakshinamurti K, Packer S, et al: Sympathetic stimulation and hypertension in the pyridoxine-deficient adult rat. Hypertension 1988;11:387–391

18 Dakshinamurti K, Paulose CS: Central nervous system origin of hypertension in the vitamin B_6 deficient adult rat; in Leklem JE, Reynolds RD (eds): Clinical and Physiological Applications of Vitamin B_6. New York, Liss, 1988, pp 159–175.

19 Dakshinamurti K, Paulose CS, Siow YL: Neurobiology of pyridoxine; in Reynolds RD, Leklem JE (eds): Vitamin B_6: Its Role in Health and Disease. New York, Liss, 1985, pp 99–121.

20 Judy WV, Watanabe AM, Henry DP, et al: Sympathetic nerve activity: Role in regulation of blood pressure in the spontaneously hypertensive rat. Circ Res 1976; 38(suppl II):1121–1129.

21 Schoemig A, Dietz R, Rascher W, et al: Sympathetic vascular tone in spontaneously hypertensive rats. Klin Wochenschr 1978;56(suppl I):1131–1138.

22 Manheim P, Hallengren B, Hanson BG: Plasma noradrenaline and blood pressure in hypothyroid patients: Effect of gradual thyroxine treatment. Clin Endocrinol 1984; 20:701–707.

23 Paulose CS, Dakshinamurti K: Chronic catheterization using vascular-access-port in rats: Blood sampling with minimal stress for plasma catecholamine determination. J Neurosci Methods 1987;22:141–146.

24 Brodie BB, Costa E, Dlabac A, et al: Application of steady state kinetics to the estimation of synthesis rate and turnover time of tissue catecholamines. J Pharmacol Exp Ther 1966;154:493–498.

25 Kobinger W, Pichler L: Relation between central sympatho-inhibitory and peripheral pre- and post-synaptic α-adrenoreceptors as evaluated by different clonidine-like substances in the rat. Naunyn-Schmiedebergs Arch Pharmacol 1980;315:21–27.

26 Sripanidkulchai B, Wyss JM: The development of α_2-adrenoceptors in the rat kidney: Correlation with noradrenergic innervation. Brain Res 1987;400:91–100.

27 Paulose CS, Dakshinamurti K: Effect of pyridoxine deficiency in young rats on high affinity serotonin and dopamine receptors. J Neurosci Res 1985;14:263–270.

28 Viswanathan M, Paulose CS, Lal KJ, et al: Alterations in brainstem α_2 adrenoreceptor activity in pyridoxine-deficient rat model of hypertension. Neurosci Lett 1990; 111:201–205.

29 DeJong W, Nukamp FP, Ohns B: Role of noradrenaline and serotonin in the control of blood pressure in normotensive and spontaneously hypertensive rats. Arch Int Pharmacodyn 1975;213:275–284.

30 Nomura M, Ohtsuji M, Nagata Y: Changes in the alpha-adrenoceptors in the medulla oblongata including nucleus tractus solitarii of spontaneously hypertensive rats. Neurochem Res 1985;10:1143–1154.

31   Rappaport A, Sturtz F, Guicheney P: Regulation of central α-adrenoreceptor by serotonergic denervation. Brain Res 1985;344:158–161.

32   Brunello N, Barbaccia ML, Chuang DM, et al: Down-regulation of β-adrenergic receptors following repeated injections of desmethylimipramine: Permissive role of serotonergic axons. Neuropharmacology 1982;21:1145–1149.

33   Bhargava KP, Tangri KK: The central vasomotor effects of 5-hydroxytryptamine. Br J Pharmacol 1959;14:411–414.

34   Smit JFM, Essen H, Struyker-Boudier HAJ: Serotonin-mediated cardiovascular responses to electric stimulation of raphe nuclei in the rat. Life Sci 1978;23:173–178.

35   Dalton DW: The cardiovascular effects of centrally administered 5-hydroxytryptamine in the conscious normotensive and hypertensive rat. J Auton Pharmacol 1986;6:67–75.

36   Wolf WA, Kuhn DM, Lovenberg W: Serotonin and central regulation of arterial blood pressure; in Vanhoutte PM (ed): Serotonin and the Cardiovascular System. New York, Raven Press, 1985, pp 63–73.

37   Peroutka SJ, Snyder SH: Multiple serotonin receptors: Differential binding of [^{3}H]5-hydroxytryptamine, [^{3}H]lysergic acid diethylamide and [^{3}H]spiroperidol. Mol Pharmacol 1979;16:687–699.

38   Martin LL, Sanders-Bush E: Comparison of the pharmacological characteristics of 5-HT$_1$ and 5-T$_2$ binding sites with those of serotonin autoreceptors which modulate serotonin release. Naunyn-Schmiedebergs Arch Pharmacol 1982;321:165–170.

39   Kalkman HO, Boddeke HWG, Doods HN, et al: Hypotensive activity of serotonin receptor agonists in rats is related to their affinity for 5-HT$_1$ receptors. Eur J Pharmacol 1983;91:155–156.

40   Leysen JE, Niemegeers CJE, Van Nueten JM, et al: Ketanserin (R41468), a selective ^{3}H-ligand of serotonin$_2$ receptor binding sites: Binding properties, brain distribution and function role. Mol Pharmacol 1982;21:301–314.

41   Saxena PR, Bolt GR, Dhasmana KM: Serotonin agonists and antagonists in experimental hypertension. J Cardiovasc Pharmacol 1987;10(suppl 3):S12–S18.

42   Saxena PR: Cardiovascular effects from stimulation of 5-hydroxytryptamine receptors. Fundam Clin Pharmacol 1989;3:245–265.

43   Wouters W, Hartog J, Bevan P: Flesinoxan. Cardiovasc Drug Rev 1988;6:71–83.

44   Kuhn DM, Wolf WA, Lovenberg W: Review of the role of central serotonergic neuronal system in blood pressure regulation. Hypertension 1980;2:243–255.

45   Fozard JR, Mir AK, Middlemise DN: Cardiovascular response to 8-hydroxy-2(di-n-propylamino) Tetralin (8-OH-DPAT) in the rat: Site of action and pharmacological analysis. J Cardiovasc Pharmacol 1987;9:328–347.

46   McCall RB, Harris LT: Role of serotonin receptor subtypes in the central regulation of blood pressure; in Rech RH, Gudelsky GA (eds): 5-HT Agonists as Psychoactive Drugs. Ann Arbor, NPP Books, 1988, pp 143–162.

47   Philippu A, Pyzuntek H, Rosensberg W: Superfusion of the hypothalamus with gamma-aminobutyric acid. Naunyn-Schmiedebergs Arch Pharmacol 1973;276:103–118.

48   Baum T, Becker FT: Hypotensive and postural effects of the γ-aminobutyric acid agonist muscimol and of clonidine. J Cardiovasc Pharmacol 1982;4:165–169.

49   Unger T, Becker H, Dietz R, et al: Antihypertensive effect of the GABA receptor

agonist muscimol in spontaneously hypertensive rats: Role of the sympathoadrenal axis. Circ Res 1984;54:30–37.

50   Persson B: Cardiovascular effects of intracerebroventricular GABA, glycine and muscimol in the rat. Naunyn-Schmiedebergs Arch Pharmacol 1980;313:225–236.

51   Persson B: GABAergic mechanisms in blood pressure control. Acta Physiol Scand 1980;(suppl 491):1–54.

52   Bhalla RC, Webb RC, Singh D: Calcium fluxes, calcium binding and adenosine cyclic 3′,5′-monophosphate-dependent protein kinase activity in the aorta of spontaneously hypertensive Kyoto-Wistar and normotensive rats. Mol Pharmacol 1978; 14:468–477.

53   Shibata S, Kuchii M, Taniguchi T: Calcium flux and binding in the aortic smooth muscle from the spontaneously hypertensive rat. Blood Vessels 1975;12:279–289.

54   Rapp JP, Nghiem CX, Oniwochei MO: Aortic calcium uptake and efflux in spontaneously hypertensive and inbred Dahl rats. J Hypertens 1986;4:493–499.

55   Shiffman FH, Bose R: A role of calcium in altered sodium ion transport of hypertensives. Life Sci 1988;42:1573–1581.

56   Viswanathan M, Bose R, Dakshinamurti K: Increased calcium influx in caudal artery of rats made hypertensive with pyridoxine deficiency. Am J Hypertens 1991; 4:252–255.

57   Noon JP, Rice PJ, Baldessarini R: Calcium leakage as a cause of the high resting tension in vascular smooth muscle from the spontaneously hypertensive rat. Proc Natl Acad Sci USA 1978;75:1605–1607.

58   Ayachi S: Increased dietary calcium lowers blood pressure in the spontaneously hypertensive rat. Metabolism 1979;28:1234–1238.

59   McCarron DA, Yung NN, Ugorety A: Disturbances of calcium metabolism in the spontaneously hypertensive rat. Hypertension 1981;3(suppl 1):I-162–I-167.

60   Lyle RM, Melby CL, Hyner GC, et al: Blood pressure and metabolic effects of calcium supplementation in normotensive whites and blacks. JAMA 1987;257: 1772–1776.

61   McCarron DA, Morris CD: Blood pressure response to oral calcium in mild to moderate hypertension: A randomized, double-blind, placebo-controlled cross-over trial. Ann Intern Med 1985;103:825–831.

62   Schleiffer R, Pernot F, Bertholet A, et al: Low calcium diet enhances the development of hypertension in the spontaneously hypertensive rat. Clin Exp Hypertens 1984;6:783–793.

63   Contley LK, Russel J, Lettieri D, et al: 1,25-Dihydroxyvitamin D_3 suppresses PTH secretion from bovine parathyroid cells in tissue culture. Endocrinology 1985;117: 2114–2119.

64   Schroeder HA: Relation between mortality from cardiovascular disease and treated water supplies. JAMA 1960;172:1902–1908.

65   Stit FW, Crawford MD, Clayton DG, et al: Clinical and biochemical indicators of cardiovascular disease among men living in hard and soft water areas. Lancet 1973; i:122–126.

66   McCarron DA, Morris CD, Henry HJ, et al: Blood pressure and nutrient intake in the United States. Science 1984;224:1392–1398.

67   Harlan WR, Hull AL, Schmonder RL, et al: Blood pressure and nutrition in adults. Am J Epidemiol 1984;120:17–28.

68   Resnick LM, Laragh JH: The hypotensive effect of short-term oral calcium loading in essential hypertension (abstract). Clin Res 1983;31:334A.

69   Belizan JM, Villar J, Pineda O, et al: Reduction of blood pressure with calcium supplementation in young adults. JAMA 1983;249:1161–1165.

70   McCarron DA: Calcium metabolism and hypertension. Kidney Int 1989;35:717–736.

71   Witteman JCM, Willet WC, Stampfer MJ, et al: Dietary calcium and magnesium and hypertension: A prospective study. Circulation 1987;76(suppl IV):35.

72   Slatopolsky E, Martin K, Morrissey J, et al: Current concepts of the metabolism and radioimmunoassay of parathyroid hormone. J Lab Clin Med 1982;99:309–316.

73   McCarron DA: Low serum concentrations of ionized calcium in patients with hypertension. N Engl J Med 1982;307:226–228.

74   Kaplan NM, Meese RB: The calcium deficiency hypothesis of hypertension: A critique. Ann Intern Med 1986;105:947–955.

75   McCarron DA: Is calcium more important than sodium in the pathogenesis of essential hypertension? Hypertension 1985;7:607–627.

76   Karanja N, McCarron DA: Calcium and hypertension. Annu Rev Nutr 1986;6:475–494.

77   Schedl HP, Miller DL, Pape JM, et al: Calcium and sodium-transport and vitamin D metabolism in the spontaneously hypertensive rat. J Clin Invest 1984;73:980–986.

78   Wright GL, Rankin GO: Concentrations of ionic and total calcium in plasma of four models of hypertension. Am J Physiol 1982;243:H365–H370.

79   Kawashima H: Altered vitamin D metabolism in the kidney of the spontaneously hypertensive rat. Biochem J 1986;237:893–897.

80   Lucas PA, Brown RC, Driicke T, et al: Abnormal vitamin D metabolism, intestinal calcium transport and bone status in the spontaneously hypertensive rat compared with its genetic control. J Clin Invest 1986;78:221–227.

81   Young EW, Patel SR, Hsu CH: Plasma $1,25(OH)_2D_3$ response to parathyroid hormone, cyclic adenosine monophosphate and phosphorous depletion in the spontaneously hypertensive rat. J Lab Clin Med 1986;108:562–566.

82   Hsu CH, Patel S, Young EW: Calcemic response to parathyroid hormone in spontaneously hypertensive rats: Role of calcitriol. J Lab Clin Med 1987;110:682–689.

83   Resnick LM: Dietary calcium and hypertension. J Nutr 1987;117:1806–1808.

84   Kurtz TW, Morris RC: Dietary intake of vitamin D as a determinant of deoxycorticosterone hypertension (abstract). Hypertension 1986;8:833.

85   Bukoski RD, McCarron DA: Altered aortic reactivity and lowered blood pressure associated with high Ca^{2+} intake in the SHR. Am J Physiol 1986;251:H976–H983.

86   Kowarski S, Cowen LA, Schachter D: Decreased content of integral membrane calcium-binding protein (IMCAL) in tissues of the spontaneously hypertensive rat. Proc Natl Acad Sci USA 1986;83:1097–1100.

87   Bukoski RD, Xue H, De Wan P, et al: Calcitropic hormones and vascular calcium metabolism in experimental hypertension; in Halpern W, et al (eds): 2nd Int Symp: Resistance Arteries. Ithaca, Perinatology Press, 1988, pp 320–328.

88   MacCarthy EP, Yamashita W, Hsu A, et al: 1,25-Dihydroxyvitamin D_3 and rat vascular smooth muscle cell growth. Hypertension 1989;13:954–959.

89 Lind L, Wengle BO, Junghall S: Blood pressure is lowered by vitamin D (alphacal-
    cidol) during long term treatment of patients with intermittent hypercalcaemia. Acta
    Med Scand 1987;222:423–427.

90 Lind L, Lithell H, Skarfors E, et al: Reduction of blood pressure by treatment with
    alphacalcidol. Acta Med Scand 1988;223:211–217.

91 Huruwitz L, McGuffe LJ, Smith PM: Specific inhibition of calcium channels by
    calcium ions in smooth muscle. J Pharmacol Exp Ther 1982;220:382–388.

92 Lind L, Wengle BO, Wide L: Hypertension in primary hyperparathyroidism: Reduc-
    tion of blood pressure by long-term treatment with vitamin D (alphacalcidol). A
    double-blind, placebo-controlled study. Am J Hypertens 1988;1:397–402.

93 Wickins D, Wilkins M, Juneo J, et al: Free-radical oxidation (peroxidation) products
    in plasma in normal and abnormal pregnancy. Ann Clin Biochem 1981;18:158–
    162.

94 Kagan VE: Lipid peroxidation in biomembranes. Boca Raton, CRC Press, 1988, pp
    119–146.

95 Hennig B, Boissonneault GA, Chow CK, et al: Effect of vitamin E on linoleic acid-
    mediated induction of peroxisomal enzymes in cultured porcine endothelial cells. J
    Nutr 1990;120:331–337.

96 Dormandy T: Free-radical oxidation and antioxidants. Lancet 1978;i:647–650.

97 Slater TF: Free radical mechanisms in tissue injury. Biochem J 1984;222:1–15.

98 Shohet SB, Pitt J, Bachner RL, et al: Lipid peroxidaiton in the killing of phagocy-
    tized pneumococci. Infect Immun 1974;10:1321–1328.

99 Johnston RB, Keele BB, Misra HP, et al: The role of superoxide anion generation in
    phagocytic bactericidal activity. J Clin Invest 1975;55:1357–1372.

100 Barrowcliffe TW, Gutteridge JM, Dormandy TL: The effect of fatty-acid autoxida-
    tion products on blood coagulation. Thromb Diath Haemorrh 1975;33:271–277.

101 Halliwell B: Oxidants in human disease: Some new concepts. FASEB J 1987;1:358–
    364.

102 Machlin LJ, Bendich A: Free radical tissue damage: Protective role of antioxidant
    nutrients. FASEB J 1987;1:441–445.

103 Lucy TA: Functional and structural aspects of biomembranes: A suggested structural
    role of vitamin E in the control of membrane permeability and stability. Ann NY
    Acad Sci 1972;203:4–16.

104 Glasuddin ASM, Diplock AT: The influence of vitamin E on membrane lipids and
    mouse fibroblasts in culture. Arch Biochem Biophys 1981;210:348–352.

105 Erin AN, Spirin MM, Tabidze LV, et al: Formation of α-tocopherol complex with
    fatty acids: A hypothetical mechanism of stabilization of biomembranes by vitamin
    E. Biochim Biophys Acta 1984;774:96–102.

106 Gavino VC, Miller JS, Ikharebha SO, et al: Effect of polyunsaturated fatty acids
    and antioxidants on lipid peroxidation in tissue culture. J Lipid Res 1981;22:763–
    769.

107 Duthie GG, Wahle KWJ, James WPT: Oxidants, antioxidants and cardiovascular
    disease. Nutr Res Rev 1989;2:51–62.

108 Pickering G: Hypertension: Causes, consequences and management. London, Chur-
    chill Livingstone, 1974.

109 Dormandy JA, Hoare E, Khattab AH, et al: Prognostic significance of rheological
    and biochemical findings in patients with intermittent claudication. Br Med J 1973;
    iv:581–583.

110 Loeper J, Emerit J, Goy J: Lipid peroxidation during atherosclerosis. IRCS Med Sci 1983;11:1034–1035.

111 Hennig B, Enoch C, Chow CK: Linoleic acid hydroperoxide increases the transfer of albumin across cultured endothelial monolayers. Arch Biochem Biophys 1986;248: 353–357.

112 Hennig B, Enoch C, Chow CK: Protection by vitamin E against endothelial cell injury by linoleic acid hydroperoxides. Nutr Res 1987;7:1253–1259.

113 Yagi K: Lipid peroxides and human diseases. Chem Phys Lipids 1987;45:337– 351.

114 Uysal M, Bulur H, Sener D, et al: Lipid peroxidation in patients with essential hypertension. Int J Clin Pharmacol Ther Toxicol 1986;24:474–476.

115 Harman D: Free radical theory of aging: The free radical diseases. Age 1984;7: 111–131.

116 Moncada S, Gryglewski RJ, Bunting S, et al: A lipid peroxide inhibits the enzyme in blood vessel microsomes that generates from prostaglandin endoperoxides the substance (prostaglandin X) which prevents platelet aggregation. Prostaglandins 1976; 12:715–737.

117 Dormandy T: Biological rancidification. Lancet 1969;ii:684.

118 Dormandy T: The autoxidation of red cells. Br J Haematol 1971;20:457–461.

119 Hubel CA, Griggs KC, McLaughlin MK: Lipid peroxidation and altered vascular function in vitamin E-deficient rats. Am J Physiol 1989;256:H1539–H1545.

120 Bendich A, Gabriel E, Machlin J: Differences in vitamin E levels in tissues of the spontaneously hypertensive and Wistar-Kyoto rats. Proc Soc Exp Biol Med 1983; 172:297–300.

121 Douglas BH, Langford HG: Toxemia of pregnancy: Production of lesions in the absence of signs. Am J Obstet Gynecol 1966;95:534–537.

122 Spitz BH, Deckmyn R, Van Bree R, et al: Influence of a vitamin E-deficient diet on prostacyclin production by mesometrial triangles and aortic rings from nondiabetic and diabetic pregnant rats. Am J Obstet Gynecol 1985;151:116–120.

123 Gant NF, Daly GL, Chand S, et al: A study of angiotensin II pressor response throughout primigravid pregnancy. J Clin Invest 1973;52:2682–2689.

124 Christman CW, Wei EP, Kontos A, et al: Effects of 15-hydroperoxy-eicosatetraenoic acid (15-HPETE) on cerebral arterioles of cats. Am J Physiol 1984;247:H631– H637.

125 Winquist RJ, Bunting PB, Baskin EP, et al: Decreased endothelium-dependent relaxation in New Zealand genetic hypertensive rats. J Hypertens 1984;2:541– 545.

126 Lockette W, Otsuka Y, Carretero O: The loss of endothelium-dependent vascular relaxation in hypertension. Hypertension 1986;8(suppl II):II-61–II-66.

Krishnamurti Dakshinamurti, Department of Biochemistry and Molecular Biology, Faculty of Medicine, University of Manitoba, Winnipeg, MB R3E 0W3 (Canada)

Simopoulos AP (ed): Nutrients in the Control of Metabolic Diseases.
World Rev Nutr Diet. Basel, Karger, 1992, vol 69, pp 74–112

Long-Chain ω3 Fatty Acids Are the Most Effective Polyunsaturated Fatty Acids for Dietary Prevention and Treatment of Cardiovascular Risk Factors

Conclusions from Clinical Studies

Peter Singer[a], Manfred Wirth[a], Ingrid Berger[a],
Brigitte Heinrich[a], Wolfgang Gödicke[a], Siegfried Voigt[a],
Christa Taube[b], Werner Jaross[c], Siegmund Gehrisch[c]

[a] Central Institute for Cardiovascular Research, Academy of Sciences, Berlin-Buch;
[b] Department of Pharmacology and Toxicology, Martin Luther University,
Halle-Wittenberg; [c] Institute of Clinical Chemistry and Laboratory Diagnostics,
Medical Academy, Dresden, FRG

Contents

Introduction 75
Slow Conversion of Linoleic and α-Linolenic Acids to Arachidonic and Eicosapen-
    taenoic Acids in Normal, Hypertensive and Hyperlipemic Subjects 75
    General Aspects 75
    Patients and Methods 77
    Results 78
    Discussion 83
Canned Mackerel as Dietary Source of Eicosapentaenoic and Docosahexaenoic
    Acids Effectively Lowers Blood Pressure, Serum Lipids, Lipoproteins and
    Thromboxane B_2 Formation in Man 84
    General Aspects 84
    Patients and Methods 86
    Results 89
    Discussion 102
Conclusion 106
References 107

Introduction

There is increasing evidence that polyunsaturated fatty acids (PUFA) on the whole exert not only a favorable effect on several risk factors of cardiovascular disease, but also that individual PUFA have different effects on blood pressure, serum lipids and lipoproteins dependent on their chemical structure (for instance, chain length and number of double bonds). Accordingly, the polyunsaturated to saturated fatty acid (P/S) ratio – which has been widely used to characterize the *quantity* of dietary PUFA in epidemiological, clinical and experimental studies – does not reflect the individual properties of different PUFA and their effects on the risk profile [1]. The discrimination between ω3 and ω6 fatty acids is becoming recognized as having pathophysiological and practical relevance, as recent clinical studies have revealed differential effects of particular PUFA types on risk factors [1–4]. This report summarizes our results from several clinical trials using vegetable oils or canned fish as various sources of dietary polyunsaturated fats. The study design was similar in several of the investigations in order to compare the results more accurately between the studies.

Slow Conversion of Linoleic and α-Linolenic Acids to Arachidonic and Eicosapentaenoic Acids in Normal, Hypertensive and Hyperlipemic Subjects

General Aspects

Previously, it had been proposed that diets enriched with linoleic acid (LA; $C_{18:2}\omega6$) or α-linolenic acid (LNA; $C_{18:3}\omega3$) stimulate the biosynthesis of eicosanoids of the 2- and 3-series, respectively, although few studies of such effect in vivo have been published.

This presumes a sufficient desaturation and elongation of LA and LNA to their C_{20}-homologue eicosanoid precursors, arachidonic acid (AA; $C_{20:4}\omega6$) and eicosapentaenoic acid (EPA; $C_{20:5}\omega3$), as a prerequisite to the proposed increase in eicosanoid formation (fig. 1). A further assumption generally made is that changes in eicosanoid formation account for the blood pressure-lowering effect of LA-rich diets in patients with essential hypertension [5–8] or in spontaneously hypertensive rats [9–11]. This hypothesis has been advanced either purely as a speculative explanation [6, 12] or based on results from laboratory animals, especially rats [7]. Only few data obtained from humans actually have demonstrated increased

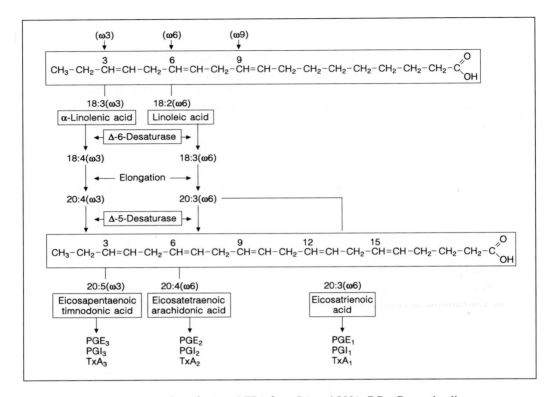

Fig. 1. Formation of AA and EPA from LA and LNA. PG = Prostaglandin.

prostaglandin metabolite excretion after LA-rich diets [13]. Furthermore, synthesis of AA from LA and, correspondingly, of EPA from LNA, which might be reflected in serum lipids from subjects ingesting, respectively, LA- and LNA-rich diets has not been convincingly demonstrated in clinical experiments. For instance, no substantial increase of EPA was seen after a diet with linseed oil (45 ml/day, equivalent to 27.0 g of LNA for 1 week) in 1 volunteer [14], but others reported a significant rise of EPA in plasma phospholipids of 10 normal subjects after an LNA-rich diet (30 ml/day of linseed oil, equivalent to 19 g of LNA for 4 weeks) [15]. A defective synthesis of AA from LA (60 ml/day of sunflowerseed oil, equivalent to 45 g of LA for 2 weeks) and of EPA from LNA (60 ml/day of linseed oil, equivalent to 38 g of LNA for 2 weeks) was proposed to exist in hypertensive patients as compared to normal subjects [16].

The extrapolation of data obtained from rats to the situation in man may be misleading, since the conversion of LA to AA and of LNA to EPA in humans is slow when compared to that in rats [9, 10]. This was considered to be due to a low activity of Δ-6-desaturase in man as a species-related defect [1, 16–19]. Consequently, the formation of eicosanoids in the human body from dietary precursors might be limited [1, 18]. To bypass this enzymatic block, PUFA-rich diets containing EPA as the direct eicosanoid precursor of the 3-series have been recommended [1, 18, 19] and, fortunately, marine oils rich in long-chain ω3 fatty acids are readily available. Corresponding dietary sources containing a high amount of long-chain ω6 fatty acids (AA), such as extracts of porcine or bovine liver, are less readily available.

In order to identify the efficacy of individual PUFA more definitely, in a series of our own clinical experiments, diets enriched with LA, LNA and EPA were given to healthy volunteers and to patients with several risk factors such as essential hypertension and primary hyperlipoproteinemia (HLP). The aim of these studies [1, 16, 20–23] was to ascertain the increase of eicosanoid precursors in serum lipids after LA-, LNA- and EPA-rich diets and to follow concomitant changes in blood pressure, serum lipids and lipoproteins.

Patients and Methods

Sixteen healthy volunteers were put on diets supplemented with either 60 ml/day of sunflowerseed oil, rich in LA (ω6), or 60 ml/day of linseed oil, rich in LNA (ω3), at 3 × 20 ml during or immediately after the main meals, over 2 weeks. Patients with mild essential hypertension (sunflowerseed oil: 10; linseed oil: 12) and subjects with primary HLP (sunflowerseed oil: 10; linseed oil: 12) underwent the same dietary regimen. From the 10 patients with HLP supplemented with sunflowerseed oil, 1 had phenotype IIa, 4 type IIb, 2 type IV and 3 type V; from the 12 hyperlipidemics on linseed-oil-rich diet, 2 had type IIa, 4 type IIb, 3 type IV and 3 type V. Pertinent clinical data of the subjects are shown in table 1.

None of the participants received any drugs. Both diets consisted of 9,000–9,300 kJ/day with a ratio of carbohydrates:fat:protein of 40:40:20 in percent kilojoules. The daily intake of LA amounted to 45 g, that of LNA to 38 g. This is probably a negligible difference from the clinical point of view. The fatty acid compositions of the oil are shown in table 2. Sodium consumption was unrestricted during the dietary periods, and body weight was unchanged. More details have been described previously [1, 2].

Before and at the end of the dietary periods, blood pressure was measured in triplicate in the recumbent and upright position by the same observer (P.S.) using the same sphygmomanometer with a standard cuff (13 × 53 cm) placed at about the midpoint of the upper arm. Diastolic blood pressure was recorded at the disappearance of Korotkoff sounds (phase 5). The values given are the means of the second and third measurements.

Table 1. Sex, age and ideal body weight within the groups studied

		Normals		Hypertensives		Hyperlipemics	
		LA (n = 16)	LNA (n = 16)	LA (n = 10)	LNA (n = 12)	LA (n = 10)	LNA (n = 12)
Sex	Female	8	8	0	0	5	5
	Male	8	8	10	12	5	7
Age, years		31 ± 10	33 ± 9	29 ± 11	29 ± 11	54 ± 11	53 ± 11
Ideal weight index, %		107 ± 10	105 ± 9	112 ± 15	109 ± 11	119 ± 13	115 ± 15

Table 2. Fatty acid composition (volume in percent) of the oils ingested

	Sunflower-seed oil	Linseed oil		Sunflower-seed oil	Linseed oil
C_{16}	4.1	3.7	$C_{18:2}\omega6$	74.7	14.5
C_{18}	2.2	2.4	$C_{18:3}\omega3$	1.4	64.0
$C_{18:1}\omega9$	14.8	14.5	$C_{20:4}\omega6$	0.1	0.2

Thereafter, blood was taken from an antecubital vein, centrifuged immediately and serum kept frozen at $-20\,°C$ until the determination of triglycerides [24], total cholesterol (enzymatically, CHOD-PAP, Boehringer-Mannheim, FRG) and fatty acid patterns of serum triglycerides, cholesterol esters and phospholipids by gas-liquid chromatography [25, 26]. High-density lipoprotein (HDL) cholesterol was estimated after precipitation with phosphotungstate and $MgCl_2$ [27]; low-density lipoprotein (LDL) cholesterol was calculated by Friedewald's formula [28]. Results are given as means ± SD. Statistical analyses were performed by the matched-pair t-test. The level of significance was accepted as p < 0.05 or p < 0.01.

Results

From figure 2 it can be seen that LA from sunflowerseed oil and LNA from linseed oil were significantly increased in serum triglycerides, cholesterol esters and phospholipids from normal subjects at the end of the dietary periods. After the LA-rich diet, however, AA remained unchanged

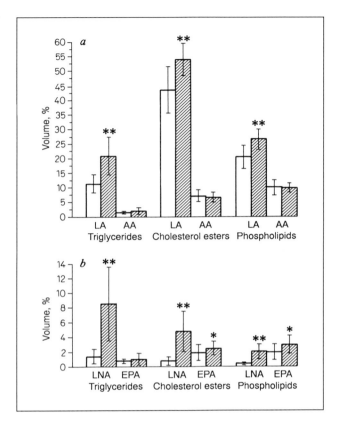

Fig. 2. Changes of LA and AA in serum lipids after an LA-rich diet (sunflowerseed oil; *a*) and of LNA and EPA after an LNA-rich diet (linseed oil; *b*) in normal subjects (n = 16). * p < 0.05; ** p < 0.01: compared to values before diet. □ = Before diet; ▨ = after diet.

within all serum lipids, whereas after the LNA-rich diet EPA appeared to increase only slightly in cholesterol esters and phospholipids. In cholesterol esters from hypertensive subjects, AA was actually lower (statistically significant) after the LA-rich diet (fig. 3). Also, patients with HLP had changed similar to those of the healthy volunteers (fig. 4), regardless of HLP phenotype.

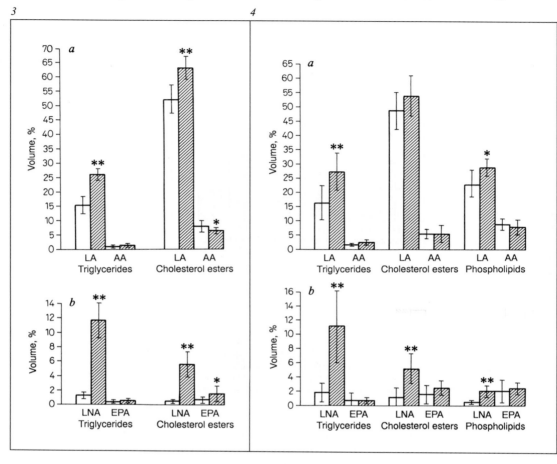

Fig. 3. Changes of LA and AA after an LA-rich diet (sunflowerseed oil; n = 10; a) and of LNA and EPA after an LNA-rich diet (linseed oil; n = 12; b) in patients with mild essential hypertension. * p < 0.05; ** p < 0.01: compared to values before diet. □ = Before diet; ▨ = after diet.

Fig. 4. Changes of LA and AA after an LA-rich diet (sunflowerseed oil; n = 10; a) and of LNA and EPA after an LNA-rich diet (linseed oil; n = 12; b) in patients with HLP. * p < 0.05; ** p < 0.01: compared to values before diet. □ = Before diet; ▨ = after diet.

Fig. 5. Blood pressure in normal, hypertensive and hyperlipemic subjects before (□) and after (▨) LA-rich (a) and LNA-rich (b) diets. * p < 0.05: compared to value before diet.

Fig. 6. Serum lipids and lipoproteins in normal subjects before (□) and after (▨) LA-rich (a) and LNA-rich (b) diets (n = 16). ** p < 0.01: compared to value before diet.

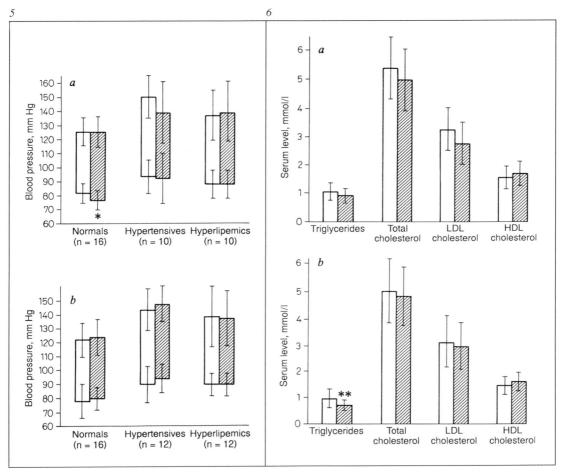

Blood pressure was unaltered in all groups studied except for the diastolic pressure in normotensive subjects (fig. 5). The clinical relevance of the latter finding remains uncertain.

Serum lipids were changed in a more different pattern. In healthy volunteers no major changes could be observed (fig. 6), while in hypertensive and hyperlipemic patients both total and LDL cholesterol were significantly lower after the LA-rich diet (fig. 7, 8). In addition, at the end of the LNA-rich diet, serum triglycerides were significantly decreased. HDL cholesterol remained unchanged in all groups studied.

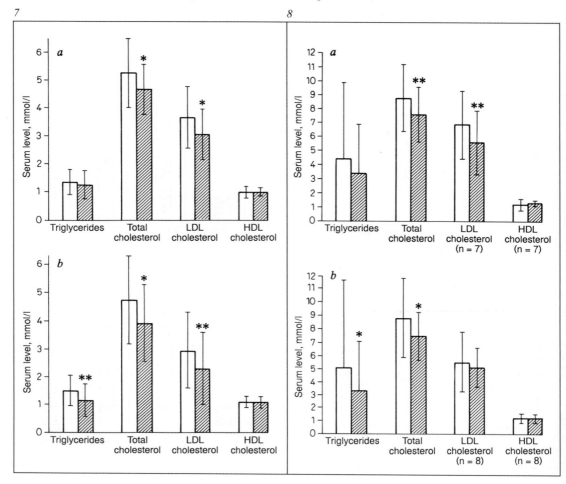

Fig. 7. Serum lipids and lipoproteins in hypertensive subjects before (□) and after
(▨) LA-rich (*a*) (n = 10) and LNA-rich (*b*) diets (n = 12). *p < 0.05; **p < 0.01:
compared to values before diet.

Fig. 8. Serum lipids and lipoproteins in hyperlipemic subjects before (□) and after
(▨) LA-rich (*a*) (n = 10) and LNA-rich (*b*) diets (n = 12). *p < 0.05; **p < 0.01:
compared to values before diet.

Discussion

Since a slow formation of AA and EPA from LA and LNA was found in normal as well as in hypertensive and hyperlipemic subjects, it is obvious that low Δ-6-desaturase activity is not directly associated with risk factors for coronary heart disease, but is a species-related feature in humans [16–19]. However, this point has been carefully studied only in short-term experiments in humans habitually ingesting high-fat diets. Intraindividual comparison in short-term and long-term studies to exclude induction of Δ-6-desaturase (with a correspondingly higher synthesis of LA to AA and LNA to EPA) by chronic intake of even smaller amounts of LA and LNA remains to be performed. In studies with longer periods of dietary intervention (6 weeks) using LA as the prevailing PUFA to significantly decrease blood pressure, the fatty acid composition of serum lipids was not measured [5, 29]. It is not yet known whether the dosage of LA and LNA, or the duration of their intake, is more important for their respective conversion to AA and EPA. Furthermore, one should keep in mind that the fatty acid pattern of serum lipids does not necessarily reflect the composition in tissues [30]. It could be speculated that the unchanged blood pressure in our short-term experiments is a result of slow formation of eicosanoid precursors and, consequently, of eicosanoids. The defective desaturation and elongation of ω3 and ω6 C_{18} fatty acids in the human body might provide a rational basis for preferring PUFA-rich diets supplemented with fish or fish oil as a source of EPA [1, 31][1]. In contrast to the blood pressure, serum lipids in hyperlipemic and hypertensive subjects were significantly influenced even by short-term intake of high amounts of LA and LNA.

This suggests that dietary LA and LNA might decrease serum lipids in a manner unrelated to the formation of eicosanoid precursors and eicosanoids. The mode of hyperlipidemic action of PUFA has been reviewed [4, 37]. However, contrary to the results obtained by EPA-rich diets (see next section), the decline of serum lipids and lipoproteins after LA- and LNA-rich diets was less pronounced, despite an approximately 20-fold higher dose (on a gram per day basis) of LA and LNA as compared to EPA.

---

[1] The obvious consequence to increase also the dietary intake of γ-linolenic acid (GLA, $C_{18:3}$ω6) in order to bypass the low Δ-6-desaturase activity [1, 16–19] will not be considered here, since the discussion is based on our own clinical experiments.

Comparative studies with LA-rich vegetable oils and EPA-rich fish oil suggest that the latter is more effective in lowering serum lipids, lipoproteins and blood pressure [3, 32, 33].

A number of studies have indicated that the efficacy of the two dietary fatty acids with C_{18} chain length, LA ($\omega 6$) and LNA ($\omega 3$), on blood pressure as well as on total and LDL cholesterol is quantitatively similar, although the latter also significantly lowers serum triglycerides [1, 2]. In view of the above, the biological effects of an $\omega 6$ C_{18} fatty acid (vegetable oil) cannot be compared with $\omega 3$ C_{20} or C_{22} fatty acids (fish oil) because of the slow conversion of C_{18} fatty acids (LA and LNA) into their C_{20} homologues (AA and EPA) based on the low activity of Δ-6-desaturase in humans. Accordingly, it cannot be determined whether the lower efficacy of vegetable oil is due to LA itself or to its slow conversion into AA and, consequently, to the slow formation of eicosanoids of the 2-series. Therefore, it seems more reliable to compare the effects of $\omega 6$ with $\omega 3$ C_{18} fatty acids (for instance, sunflowerseed oil rich in LA with linseed oil rich in LNA) or $\omega 3$ C_{18} fatty acids (i.e. LNA) with $\omega 3$ C_{20} fatty acids (i.e. EPA). This has been performed recently [1], finding qualitative differences between LA and LNA, but qualitative and quantitative differences between LNA and EPA. [A comparison of an $\omega 6$ C_{18} fatty acid (LA) with an $\omega 6$ C_{20} fatty acid (AA) is not possible from the dietetic point of view, since a nutrient source rich in AA is not readily available.] Consequently, not only the $\omega 3$ or $\omega 6$ positions of the first double bond or the degree of unsaturation, but also the chain length of PUFA is important for its physiological effects.

Canned Mackerel as Dietary Source of Eicosapentaenoic and Docosahexaenoic Acids Effectively Lowers Blood Pressure, Serum Lipids, Lipoproteins and Thromboxane B_2 Formation in Man

General Aspects

If PUFA effects are via alterations in eicosanoid synthesis, it seems reasonable to prefer EPA-rich diets in order to bypass the enzymatic block at the Δ-6-desaturase level (fig. 9). Based on this suggestion, a higher efficacy of EPA-rich diets could be anticipated.

Diets supplemented with EPA-rich fish or fish oil have been described to lower effectively serum triglycerides, total and LDL cholesterol in normolipemic [34, 35] and hyperlipemic [31, 36] subjects. On the other hand, some clinical experiments using dietary $\omega 3$ fatty acids have found an

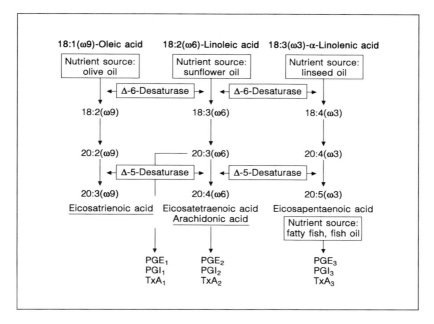

Fig. 9. Position of EPA in the PUFA system, its nutrient sources and conversion to prostaglandin (PG) precursors.

increase of LDL cholesterol [37]. Despite this finding, a significantly reduced restenosis rate was found after coronary angioplasty [38]. In some of the studies, HDL cholesterol appeared to be increased [34, 35], but unchanged in others [32, 39]. Blood pressure measurements performed in normotensive volunteers showed a decrease in systolic and diastolic [20, 40] or only systolic [32, 41] values within the normal range. Subsequently, a blood pressure-lowering effect was also described in patients with mild essential hypertension [21, 23, 42, 43]. The overall conclusion from the existing data is that marine fish and fish products exert a beneficial effect on several risk factors for atherosclerosis.

We used canned mackerel in a commercially available form as an alternative dietary source of EPA. This might be a more appropriate reflection of the nutritional habits (tendency to fast foods) in populations of industrialized countries than would be their supplementation with fresh fish or fish oil. The aim of the studies was to evaluate the effects of a mackerel diet on blood pressure, serum lipids and lipoproteins in healthy volunteers and in several risk groups under the same experimental conditions. Furthermore, a practical dietary regimen was tested in a long-term trial in patients with mild essential hypertension.

Patients and Methods

In 3 of the studies the subjects received 2 cans daily of commercially available mackerel or herring fillet in tomato pulp for 2 weeks, in a crossover design. The fat content and fatty acid composition of fish flesh (140 g/can) and pulp (70 g/can) have been described previously in detail [18]. In short, the amount of EPA ingested was 1.1 g/can or 2.2 g daily in the mackerel period and 0.5 g/can or 1.0 g daily in the herring period, which served as a control. The corresponding amounts of docosahexaenoic acid (DHA; $C_{22:6}\omega3$) were 2.8 g/day during the mackerel period and 1.8 g/day during the herring diet. Sodium and potassium contents of canned mackerel were slightly higher (1.4 and 0.9 g/can, respectively) than those of herring (1.1 and 0.8 g/can, respectively). The mean energy intake amounted to 9,000–9,800 kJ/day (40% carbohydrates, 40% fat and 20% protein) without major differences between the dietary periods. In both isocaloric periods, the qualitative composition of food was equal, only the species of fish changed. The participants were requested to maintain their normal physical activities and nutritional habits, but to omit cold cuts of their own choice and, thereby, to reduce their daily fat intake by nearly 50 g in order to balance the energy provided by the canned fish (1,200 kJ/can). Fluids were allowed ad libitum, the subjects being asked to avoid excessive alcohol and to omit it on the day before blood sampling. Usually, the content of one can was eaten in the late morning, the other in the evening. The sodium intake was unrestricted during the dietary periods, and the protocols revealed no significant deviations during the dietary periods or during the interval on normal food. No complaints were reported during the diets and none of the subjects dropped out.

Study 1. Fifteeen healthy volunteers (10 males, 5 females), receiving no medication, were given the diets described. Their mean age was 37.5 ± 5.5 (SD) years and their ideal body weight index was 1.09 ± 0.09. Body weight remained constant during the study. In 10 subjects the mackerel period preceded the herring period with an interval of 3 months on normal food (washout). In 5 subjects the sequence was reversed (fig. 10). The beginning of the second period corresponded to the control after the first period. Controls of the second period were performed 3 months later.

Before and at the end of each dietary period, as well as 3 months after the second period, blood pressure was measured in triplicate in the recumbent position. Venous blood was taken from an antecubital vein, immediately centrifuged and serum kept frozen at $-20\,°C$ until the determination of triglyerides, total and LDL cholesterol, HDL cholesterol, dopamine β-hydroxylase activity [44] as well as the fatty acid patterns of triglycerides and cholesterol esters by gas-liquid chromatography using the methods described in the preceding section. For the radioenzymatic assay of catecholamines [45], heparinized plasma was used.

Study 2. Fourteen male patients with mild essential hypertension (diastolic blood pressure 90–104 mm Hg), all of them being normolipemic nonsmokers and receiving no

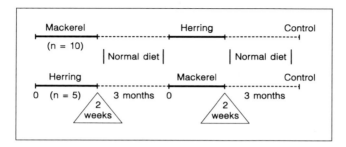

Fig. 10. Study design of crossover experiments in healthy volunteers (study 1). The same design was used in patients with mild essential hypertension (study 2) and HPL (study 3).

drugs, were put on the same diets (compare study 1). The diagnosis of essential hypertension was based on physical examination, ECG, X-ray and extensive laboratory studies to exclude secondary hypertension. The mean age of the patients was 35.3 ± 6.0 years (mean $\pm$ SD) and their ideal body weight index was 1.13 ± 0.11. In 8 patients canned mackerel was supplemented in the first dietary period; in 6 subjects canned herring was given initially. Before and after 2 weeks of diet, as well as 3 months after the second period, blood pressure was measured 3 times in the recumbent and upright position. Thereafter, blood was withdrawn for determination of the same parameters as in study 1, including the fatty acid pattern of phospholipids. Before and 30, 60 and 120 min after a standardized oral glucose load (75 g), capillary blood was taken from the earlobe for glucose determination [46], and venous blood was withdrawn via an indwelling catheter for the estimation of plasma free fatty acids [47] and insulin (ROTOP Radioimmuno-Test) [48]. At least 1 h later a psychophysiological stress test (mental arithmetics, sentence completion tasks) was carried out [49]. After a 20-min period of rest immediately before the test, and during the sentence completion tasks plasma catecholamines [45] and plasma thromboxane B_2 (TxB_2) [21, 50] were estimated.

Study 3. Fifteen patients (7 males, 8 females) with primary HLP (2 phenotype IIa, 5 type IIb, 3 type IV and 5 type V) – 10 of them without medication and 5 receiving drugs without known influence on lipid metabolism – were put on the isocaloric diets described. The mean age of the subjects was 54 ± 11 years and the ideal body weight index was 1.15 ± 0.14. No other relevant diseases except mild arterial hypertension in 9 of the cases were known. The diagnosis of primary HLP was based on the exclusion of diseases leading to secondary HLP. For phenotyping [51] the levels of serum triglycerides, total and LDL cholesterol as well as chylomicron tests showed unequivocal results. In 8 of the patients the mackerel period preceded the herring diet; in 7 patients the herring diet came first.

Blood pressure measurement and blood sampling were performed as described for study 2. HDL and LDL cholesterol were calculated in 9 patients with initial triglyceride levels below 4.5 mmol/l. In addition, apolipoproteins AI, B, CII and CIII were determined by electroimmunoassay [52, 53].

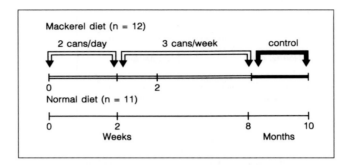

Fig. 11. Study design comparing a high-dose short-term period (2 weeks) providing 2 cans of mackerel/day with a low-dose long-term period (8 months) providing 3 cans of mackerel/week in patients with mild essential hypertension (study 4).

Study 4. Twelve untreated male patients with mild essential hypertension were put on diets of various duration supplemented with different amounts of canned mackerel. Their mean age was 32.8 ± 9.1 years and the ideal body weight index was 1.14 ± 0.15. Eleven male mildly hypertensive subjects matched for age, body weight index, blood pressure and serum lipids, continuing their nutritional habits, served as controls. Their mean age was 36.1 ± 5.9 years and the body weight index was 1.13 ± 0.07.

In the first (short-term) period of 2 weeks the patients of the dietary group received 2 cans/day of mackerel in tomato pulp corresponding to the mackerel diet in studies 1 through 3. The consignment of the cans (commercially available mackerel fillet in tomato pulp), was a single purchase of one batch prior to the start of the trial. During the second (long-term) period of 8 months, 3 cans/week of mackerel were ingested by the same individuals. All of the other conditions were similar to the first dietary period. The intake of EPA and DHA in the long-term period amounted to 3.3 and 4.2 g/week corresponding to 0.5 g/day and 0.6 g/day , respectively. During the third period of 2 months (control), the patients returned to their dietary habits prior to the trial (fig. 11). There were no major deviations in energy uptake from the other dietary periods. Body weight remained constant during the study. The 11 control subjects continued their normal diets and physical activities throughout the experiment. Energy, fat and cholesterol intake were similar in both groups of hypertensive patients.

Before and at the end of each dietary period, blood pressure in the recumbent position was measured 3 times in the early morning under the conditions described for the preceding studies. During the second period an additional measurement 2 months after its beginning was carried out in the dietary group (compliance control). Blood was withdrawn from an antecubital vein after an overnight fast for the estimation of serum lipids and lipoproteins (compare study 1) and serum sodium and potassium with a flame photometer (FLM 3/Radiometer, Copenhagen, Denmark).

Six milliliters of blood were allowed to clot in a water bath (37 °C) for 1 h and then centrifuged at 5,000 rpm [54]. Serum was kept frozen till the estimation of TxB_2, the

Table 3. Selected fatty acids of serum triglycerides and cholesterol esters (mean ± SD of volume in percent) from healthy subjects before and after a mackerel or herring diet

Fatty acids	Mackerel diet		Herring diet	
	before	after	before	after
Serum triglycerides				
$C_{18:2}\omega6$	13.8 ± 4.0	11.8 ± 2.2	14.6 ± 4.3	14.7 ± 4.0
$C_{20:4}\omega6$	1.4 ± 0.5	2.1 ± 0.5**	1.5 ± 0.4	2.1 ± 0.9
$C_{20:5}\omega3$	0.4 ± 1.0	2.1 ± 1.1**	0.2 ± 0.3	0.3 ± 0.3
$C_{22:6}\omega3$	0.6 ± 0.5	6.7 ± 4.7**	1.3 ± 0.5	7.6 ± 2.7**
P/S ratio	0.68 ± 0.24	1.03 ± 0.35*	0.71 ± 0.20	1.19 ± 0.28**
$C_{20:5}/C_{20:4}$	0.29 ± 0.05	0.98 ± 0.46**	0.13 ± 0.14	0.15 ± 0.24
Cholesterol esters				
$C_{18:2}\omega6$	49.9 ± 6.0	39.8 ± 4.1**	52.1 ± 5.4	46.7 ± 5.5**
$C_{20:4}\omega6$	8.1 ± 3.3	8.0 ± 0.9	7.2 ± 1.5	7.3 ± 0.9
$C_{20:5}\omega3$	1.5 ± 1.2	10.9 ± 2.0**	1.9 ± 1.2	8.2 ± 2.7**
$C_{22:6}\omega3$	0.7 ± 0.8	1.9 ± 0.3**	0.8 ± 0.2	1.6 ± 0.5**
P/S ratio	5.29 ± 1.18	4.54 ± 0.45	5.74 ± 0.94	5.50 ± 0.84
$C_{20:5}/C_{20:4}$	0.17 ± 0.07	1.37 ± 0.19**	0.26 ± 0.11	1.12 ± 0.29**

* $p < 0.05$; ** $p < 0.01$: significant difference between values before and after diet.
P/S ratio = Polyunsaturated to saturated fatty acid ratio.

stable metabolite of TxA_2, by radioimmunoassay after dilution with phosphate buffer at 1:1,000. The method has been described elsewhere [50]. Urine volume as well as urinary excretion of sodium and potassium by flame photometry (FLM 3), vanillylmandelic acid [55], adrenaline and noradrenaline after the modified method of von Euler and Lishajko [56] were estimated from a sample of the 24-hour period prior to the day of blood sampling.

All results are given as mean ± SD. Statistical analyses of the data before versus after the diets, as well as versus the washout period, were performed by the matched-pair t-test, the level of significance being accepted as $p < 0.05$ or $p < 0.01$.

Results

Study 1. As can be seen from table 3, EPA and DHA were significantly augmented in serum lipids, the former appearing more in cholesterol esters and the latter more in triglycerides. The increase of EPA and of the ratio of EPA to AA was more pronounced after the mackerel diet according to the

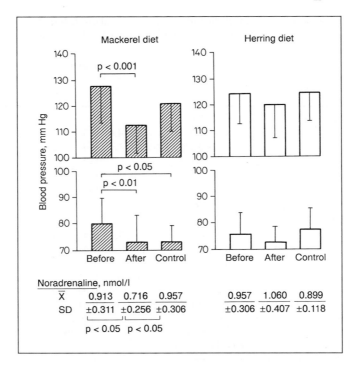

Fig. 12. Blood pressure and plasma noradrenaline in healthy volunteers (n = 15) before and after a mackerel or herring diet (2 cans/day for 2 weeks), and at control (after washout) 3 months later.

higher amount of EPA ingested. Concomitantly, LA in cholesterol esters declined, whereas AA rose only in triglycerides. The polyunsaturated to saturated fatty acid (P/S) ratio was increased in serum triglycerides, but was unchanged in cholesterol esters. A similar pattern of PUFA incorporation into serum lipids was found in studies 2 and 3 (data not shown).

Systolic and diastolic blood pressure, which were within the normal range prior to the study, were significantly decreased at the end of the mackerel diet (fig. 12). Systolic blood pressure had not returned completely to baseline values 3 months later, and diastolic blood pressure remained at the lower values. After the herring-supplemented diet the blood pressure showed no alteration. Plasma noradrenaline was markedly depressed after the mackerel diet and appeared unchanged after the herring period.

Table 4. Serum lipids and lipoproteins from healthy subjects (n = 15) before and after a mackerel or herring diet, and at control 3 months later

	Before	After	Control
Mackerel diet			
Serum triglycerides	1.23 ± 0.50	$0.65 \pm 0.19**$	$1.05 \pm 0.41**$
Total cholesterol	5.26 ± 0.89	$4.87 \pm 0.95*$	$5.22 \pm 0.70*$
LDL cholesterol	3.31 ± 0.91	3.10 ± 0.89	3.38 ± 0.69
HDL cholesterol	1.38 ± 0.34	1.45 ± 0.34	1.27 ± 0.33
LDL/HDL cholesterol	2.52 ± 0.83	2.27 ± 0.83	2.80 ± 0.87
Dopamine β-hydroxylase	102 ± 44	97 ± 49	99 ± 46
Herring diet			
Serum triglycerides	0.87 ± 0.41	0.81 ± 0.40	0.99 ± 0.49
Total cholesterol	5.32 ± 0.65	5.14 ± 0.69	5.25 ± 0.57
LDL cholesterol	3.68 ± 0.69	3.39 ± 0.77	3.71 ± 0.68
HDL cholesterol	1.32 ± 0.29	1.38 ± 0.25	1.44 ± 0.34
LDL/HDL cholesterol	2.92 ± 0.94	2.59 ± 0.83	2.64 ± 0.85
Dopamine β-hydroxylase	99 ± 46	96 ± 55	84 ± 33

Lipid and lipoprotein values are expressed as millimoles per liter, and those of dopamine β-hydroxylase as international units. $* p < 0.05$; $** p < 0.01$; significant difference between values before and after diet or between values after diet and at control 3 months later.

Plasma adrenaline (not shown) and dopamine β-hydroxylase activity (table 4) did not change from baseline values throughout the study.

Serum triglycerides and total cholesterol were significantly lower at the end of the mackerel period, returning to the initial levels 3 months later (table 4). The decrease of LDL cholesterol and the increase of HDL cholesterol did not reach the level of statistical significance. After the herring diet, only minor changes were seen.

Study 2. In patients with mild essential hypertension, systolic blood pressure was significantly depressed in the recumbent (fig. 13), but not in the upright, position (data not shown) after the mackerel diet. It remained unchanged after ingesting the herring diet. Systolic and diastolic blood pressure before and during the psychophysiological stress test were markedly lowered after the mackerel period as compared to the values prior to the diet (fig. 14). But the blood pressure increment with stress was identical

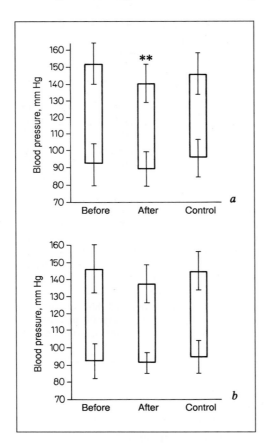

Fig. 13. Blood pressure in the recumbent position in patients with mild essential hypertension before and after a mackerel (*a*) or herring (*b*) diet, and at control 3 months later. ** p < 0.01: compared to values before diet.

on the two occasions. After the herring diet, the decrease of blood pressure was significant only immediately after the period of mental load (arithmetics, sentence completion tasks). The changes in heart rate were the same during the stress test regardless of diet. The return of the blood pressure values after the washout period was omitted in figure 14 for simplicity of presentation. Plasma noradrenaline was not markedly increased at the end of the stress test when compared with the level prior to the mental load. This might be due to the relatively mild stressors used. No difference in the patterns of plasma catecholamines was induced by the diets (data not shown). Plasma TxB_2 rose significantly during the stress test (fig. 15). After both dietary periods this increase failed to occur.

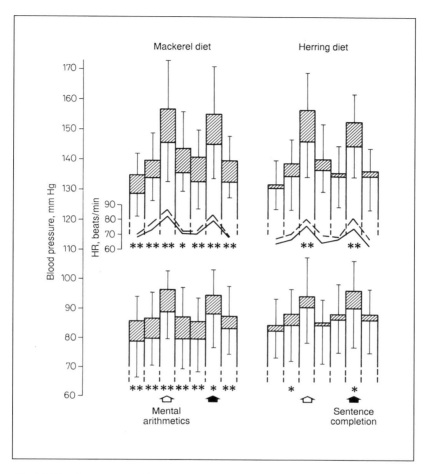

Fig. 14. Blood pressure and heart rate (HR) from patients with mild essential hypertension during a psychophysiological stress test before (□) and after (▨) a mackerel or herring diet (control 3 months later not shown). * p < 0.05; ** p < 0.01.

Serum triglycerides, total and LDL cholesterol and the LDL cholesterol to HDL cholesterol ratio were markedly depressed after the mackerel diet, whereas HDL cholesterol appeared significantly higher (table 5). Except for HDL cholesterol and the LDL cholesterol to HDL cholesterol ratio, the values had returned to the initial levels 3 months later. At the end of the herring period the changes were minor.

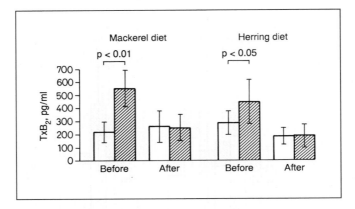

Fig. 15. TxB$_2$ formation in plasma from patients with mild essential hypertension during a psychophysiological stress test (compare fig. 14) before and after a mackerel (left side) or herring diet (right side). ☐ = before test and; ▨ = after sentence completion tasks (compare fig. 14).

Table 5. Serum lipids and lipoproteins from patients with mild essential hypertension (n = 14) before and after a mackerel or herring diet, and at control 3 months later

	Before	After	Control
Mackerel diet			
Serum triglycerides	1.26 ± 0.42	0.91 ± 0.25*	1.33 ± 0.69*
Total cholesterol	5.16 ± 0.80	4.73 ± 0.71**	5.20 ± 0.85*
LDL cholesterol	3.66 ± 0.94	3.15 ± 0.81**	3.60 ± 0.92*
HDL cholesterol	1.25 ± 0.30	1.40 ± 0.32*	1.42 ± 0.30
LDL/HDL cholesterol	3.29 ± 1.87	2.47 ± 1.21**	2.66 ± 0.93
Herring diet			
Serum triglycerides	1.23 ± 0.71	0.99 ± 0.41	1.50 ± 0.55**
Total cholesterol	4.99 ± 0.94	4.68 ± 0.81	5.06 ± 0.83
LDL cholesterol	3.46 ± 0.85	3.14 ± 1.00	3.42 ± 0.79
HDL cholesterol	1.30 ± 0.30	1.40 ± 0.36	1.34 ± 0.32
LDL/HDL cholesterol	2.87 ± 0.95	2.45 ± 1.14	2.73 ± 1.09

Values are expressed as millimoles per liter.
* $p < 0.05$; ** $p < 0.01$: significant difference between values before and after diet or between values after diet and at control 3 months later.

Study 3. In patients with HLP, serum triglycerides, total and LDL cholesterol as well as the LDL cholesterol to HDL cholesterol ratio appeared significantly lower at the end of the mackerel diet and, thereafter, returned nearly to the initial values (table 6). The changes seen after the herring period were of a minor degree. Because of the marked variability, the standard deviations (especially of serum triglycerides) were large. The decrease of triglycerides and total cholesterol at 2 weeks was more pronounced if the initial values were extraordinarily high (fig. 16, 17). On the other hand, the rise of HDL cholesterol at the end of the mackerel period did not reach statistical significance, but was significantly increased after the herring diet (table 6). During the washout periods the values returned to the initial levels. Although blood glucose and insulin during the glucose tolerance test remained unchanged after both fish diets (not shown), free fatty acids were significantly lower at the end of the mackerel period, returning to the baseline level 3 months later (fig. 18). Apolipoproteins AI and B, the former being lower and the latter being higher as compared to

Table 6. Serum lipids and lipoproteins from patients with HPL (n = 15) before and after a mackerel or herring diet, and at control 3 months later

	Before	After	Control
Mackerel diet			
Serum triglycerides	9.02 ± 8.99	3.77 ± 5.02**	6.24 ± 7.42*
Total cholesterol	9.07 ± 2.43	7.48 ± 1.77**	9.15 ± 2.39**
LDL cholesterol	6.71 ± 1.83[a]	5.26 ± 1.14**	7.01 ± 2.01**
HDL cholesterol	1.21 ± 0.19[a]	1.32 ± 0.25	1.18 ± 0.25
LDL/HDL cholesterol	5.69 ± 1.96	4.25 ± 1.58*	6.26 ± 2.80*
Herring diet			
Serum triglycerides	6.89 ± 7.26	3.40 ± 3.04*	10.24 ± 17.85
Total cholesterol	8.73 ± 2.59	8.05 ± 2.46*	9.99 ± 3.35**
LDL cholesterol	5.71 ± 2.74[a]	5.39 ± 2.18	6.42 ± 2.71
HDL cholesterol	1.16 ± 0.23[a]	1.37 ± 0.28**	1.18 ± 0.39
LDL/HDL cholesterol	5.13 ± 3.08	4.14 ± 2.09*	5.81 ± 3.48*

Values are expressed as millimoles per liter.
* $p < 0.05$; ** $p < 0.01$: significant difference between values before and after diet or between values after diet and at control 3 months later.
[a] Values from 9 subjects with serum triglycerides below 4.5 mmol/l.

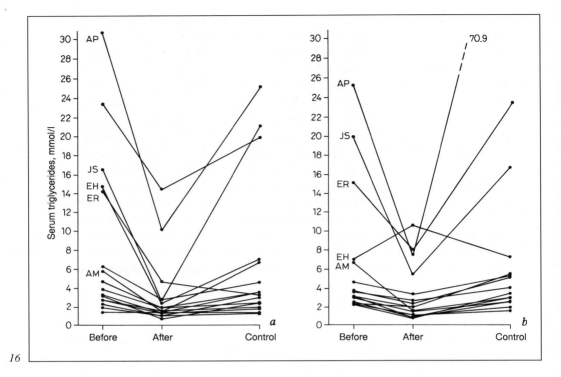

16

Fig. 16. Serum triglycerides in patients with HLP before and after a mackerel (*a*) or herring (*b*) diet, and at control 3 months later. AP, JS, EH, ER and AM = initials of some patients.

Fig. 17. Total cholesterol in patients with HLP before and after a mackerel (*a*) or herring (*b*) diet, and at control 3 months later. EH, ST, W, AP and AM = initials of some patients.

Fig. 18. Free fatty acids during an oral glucose tolerance test (75 g) in patients with HPL before (——) and after (-·-·-) a mackerel (*a*) or herring (*b*) diet, and at control 3 months later (---). *p < 0.05; ** p < 0.01.

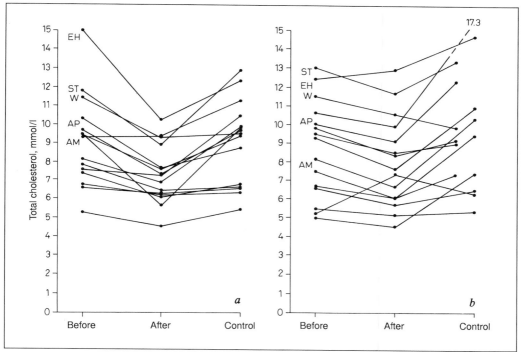

17

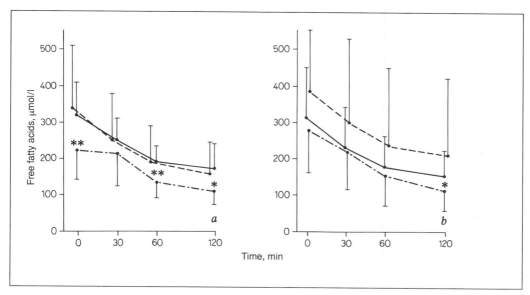

18

Table 7. Apolipoproteins AI, B, CII and CIII from patients with HPL before and after a mackerel or herring diet, and at control 3 months later

	Before	After	Control
Mackerel diet			
Apolipoprotein AI	111±41	93±33	113±17
Apolipoprotein B	285±122	271±116	264±135
Apolipoprotein CII	4.5±1.0	3.1±0.5**	4.9±1.1**
Apolipoprotein CIII	21.0±8.5	16.0±3.8*	21.2±2.5**
Herring diet			
Apolipoprotein AI	114±20	116±22	118±21
Apolipoprotein B	261±139	258±126	206±50
Apolipoprotein CII	5.5±3.0	4.4±2.4*	4.1±0.6
Apolipoprotein CIII	24.9±13.4	20.4±6.0	25.3±11.5

Values are expressed as milligrams per deciliter.
* $p < 0.05$; ** $p < 0.01$: significant difference between values before and after diet or between values after diet and at control 3 months later.

reference values of healthy subjects from our laboratory (127 ± 27 and 98 ± 24 mg/dl, respectively), were unchanged after both dietary periods (table 7). Apolipoproteins CII and CIII (reference values: 4.5 ± 3.0 and 13.5 ± 9.0 mg/dl) were significantly decreased after the mackerel diet, their ratio remaining constant. At the end of the herring period, only small changes were found. Systolic blood pressure in both the recumbent and upright position was significantly lower after the mackerel diet and had returned nearly to the initial levels at the end of the washout period (table 8). Diastolic blood pressure in the upright position was slightly decreased and appeared unchanged in the recumbent position. Both systolic and diastolic blood pressure remained unchanged after the herring diet. After division into 2 subgroups the decline of systolic blood pressure with initial values of 160 mm Hg and above was more pronounced in the recumbent as well as in the upright position after the mackerel period (table 8). Systolic blood pressure below 160 mm Hg decreased likewise, but at a low level of significance. Thus, the higher blood pressure values were decreased more obviously.

Study 4. EPA was increased in all serum lipid fractions of the hypertensive subjects on the mackerel diet (2 cans/day) at the end of the short-

Table 8. Systolic and diastolic blood pressure in the recumbent and upright position in patients with HPL (n = 15) before and after a mackerel or herring diet, and at control 3 months later

	Before	After	Control
Mackerel diet			
Recumbent			
systolic	151 ± 28	140 ± 23**	148 ± 26*
≥ 160 mm Hg (n = 6)	178 ± 17	161 ± 21**	168 ± 21
< 160 mm Hg (n = 9)	133 ± 14	126 ± 11*	133 ± 17*
diastolic	94 ± 12	91 ± 12	94 ± 13
Upright			
systolic	151 ± 27	137 ± 20**	146 ± 24*
≥ 160 mm Hg	175 ± 18	151 ± 20**	163 ± 16
< 160 mm Hg	130 ± 11	125 ± 9*	130 ± 20
diastolic	101 ± 13	93 ± 10*	98 ± 10*
Herring diet			
Recumbent			
systolic	150 ± 22	145 ± 25	146 ± 24
diastolic	95 ± 12	92 ± 13	96 ± 18
Upright			
systolic	147 ± 23	145 ± 28	145 ± 24
diastolic	99 ± 9	97 ± 12	98 ± 13

Values are expressed as millimeters mercury.
* $p < 0.05$; ** $p < 0.01$: significant difference between values before and after diet or between values after diet and at control 3 months later.

term period of 2 weeks (fig. 19). The most pronounced increase occurred in the cholesterol esters. During the long-term period (8 months) providing a lower dose of EPA (3 cans/week of mackerel), this fatty acid declined in serum lipids and after 8 months reached values which were only twice as high as the basal levels. After the washout period, values had returned to the initial levels. In the control group no statistically significant changes were found.

Systolic and diastolic blood pressure were significantly lower at the end of the short-term dietary period (fig. 20). In the subsequent long-term period it remained at reduced values, only returning to the baseline levels at the end of the washout period. In the control group the initial blood

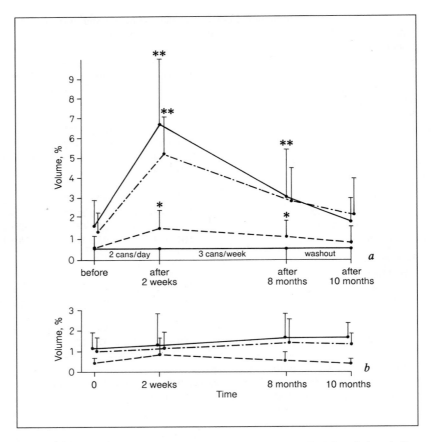

Fig. 19. EPA in serum triglycerides (– – –), cholesterol esters (——) and phospholip-ids (·····) from patients with mild essential hypertension before and after a high-dose short-term (2 cans/day for 2 weeks) and a low-dose long-term (3 cans/week for 8 months) mackerel diet and at control (after washout) 2 months later. *a* Mackerel diet. * $p < 0.05$; ** $p < 0.05$. *b* Group on normal diet.

pressure was slightly lower when compared with the mackerel group and showed no alteration during the trial.

Serum triglycerides, total and LDL cholesterol, and the LDL choles-terol to HDL cholesterol ratio appeared significantly decreased at the end of the short-term period (table 9). Two and 8 months later (during and at the end of the long-term period), the triglyceride level increased back to a

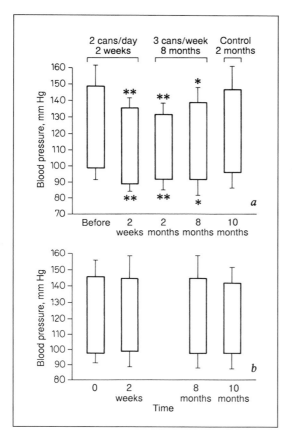

Fig. 20. Blood pressure of patients with mild essential hypertension before and after a high-dose short-term (2 cans/day for 2 weeks) and a low-dose long-term (3 cans/week for 8 month) mackerel diet, and at control (after washout) 2 months later. *a* Mackerel diet (n = 12). * p < 0.01; ** p < 0.001. *b* Group on normal diet (n = 11).

level not significantly lower than baseline. After the washout period, it had increased further and slightly exceeded the initial values. Total and LDL cholesterol returned to the initial levels more slowly, i.e. at the end of the long-term period, and increased further until the end of the washout period. HDL cholesterol was significantly increased after the short-term period and, thereafter, returned to the baseline levels. No significant alterations of

Table 9. Serum lipids, lipoproteins and TxB_2 formation in patients with mild essential hypertension (n = 12) before and after a short-term (2 weeks, 2 cans/day) and long-term (8 months, 3 cans/week) mackerel diet as well as 2 months later (washout), and in a control group (n = 11) on normal diet

	Short-term diet		Long-term diet		Washout 2 months
	before	2 weeks	2 months	8 months	
Mackerel diet					
Serum triglycerides	1.40 ± 0.53	1.10 ± 0.46*	1.25 ± 0.57	1.29 ± 0.57	1.58 ± 0.57
Total cholesterol	5.58 ± 0.67	4.98 ± 0.41**	5.12 ± 0.99*	5.37 ± 0.93	5.65 ± 0.64
LDL cholesterol	3.90 ± 0.67	3.13 ± 0.87*	3.54 ± 0.83*	3.70 ± 1.06	4.02 ± 0.71
HDL cholesterol	1.39 ± 0.33	1.63 ± 0.59*	1.33 ± 0.37	1.42 ± 0.39	1.32 ± 0.30
LDL/HDL cholesterol	2.71 ± 0.89	2.04 ± 1.01**	2.57 ± 0.70	2.67 ± 1.31	3.05 ± 1.56
Thromboxane B_2	140 ± 79	61 ± 33**	105 ± 73	161 ± 87	123 ± 113
Normal diet					
Serum triglycerides	1.36 ± 0.49	1.53 ± 0.80	–	1.51 ± 0.63	1.44 ± 0.47
Total cholesterol	6.00 ± 0.82	6.30 ± 1.24	–	5.58 ± 0.41	5.68 ± 0.41
LDL cholesterol	4.34 ± 0.60	4.58 ± 1.10	–	4.32 ± 0.40	4.12 ± 0.42
HDL cholesterol	1.39 ± 0.51	1.41 ± 0.23	–	1.23 ± 0.43	1.28 ± 0.40
LDL/HDL cholesterol	3.32 ± 1.64	3.25 ± 0.87	–	3.40 ± 1.34	3.18 ± 0.91
Thromboxane B_2	120 ± 88	205 ± 174	–	133 ± 59	189 ± 103

Lipid and lipoprotein values are expressed as millimoles per liter, those of TxB_2 as nanograms per milliliter. * $p < 0.05$; ** $p < 0.01$: significantly different from initial values.

serum lipids and lipoproteins could be found within the control group continuing its normal diet.

The formation of TxB_2 in serum was significantly lower after the short-term period in the dietary group and returned to normal thereafter (table 9). No changes were seen in the control group. Serum electrolytes, urine volume as well as the excretion of sodium, potassium, adrenaline, noradrenaline and vanillylmandelic acid showed no changes in any of the subjects (data not shown).

Discussion

In all subjects studied, the predominant incorporation of EPA into cholesterol esters and of DHA into serum triglycerides was confirmed, indicating a dissimilar metabolic fate of these two ω3 fatty acids after alimentary uptake [20, 34]. In general, during the 3 short-term studies a

2-fold higher percentage of EPA in serum lipids after the mackerel diet as compared to the herring diet could be observed. This is consistent with the 2-fold higher content of EPA in the canned mackerel. A dose-response relationship could also be seen in the long-term experiment. In addition, the increase of the ω3 fatty acids in serum lipids verified the participants' compliance. The decrease of LA in serum triglycerides (nonsignificant) and cholesterol esters (significant) and the marked increase of AA in serum triglycerides, seen in normal, hypertensive and hyperlipemic subjects [20–22], suggest a differential effect of dietary ω3 fatty acids on these two ω6 fatty acids. This might have been caused by the low dietary supply of LA during the EPA-rich diet, associated with an adaptively higher activity of Δ-6-desaturase in liver and, therefore, a higher AA content of triglycerides in very-low-density lipoprotein (VLDL) released from the liver [57]. This is consistent with an increased formation not only of prostaglandin I_3, but also of prostaglandin I_2 after diets supplemented with mackerel or fish oil [58]. The decrease of LA by dietary ω3 fatty acids can be ignored from the nutritional standpoint provided there is an abundant intake of LA as might be the case under normal conditions in industrialized countries. On the other hand, from recent experiments in rats it is known that extreme diets with exclusive feeding of cod liver oil as dietary fat lead to a dramatic fall of LA with signs of essential fatty acid deficiency [59–61]. This confirms the impression of several authors [62, 63] that, to avoid developing ω6 fatty acid deficiency in rats, one must feed some corn oil together with fish oil. From these results it can be concluded that dietary ω3 fatty acids (marine fish, fish oil) should not be considered an alternative, but a complement to ω6 PUFA (vegetable oil). Therefore, further research is needed to find the best balance between the ω3 and ω6 fatty acid supply from the nutritional point of view.

The decrease of serum triglycerides, total and LDL cholesterol was found in healthy volunteers as well as in patients with mild essential hypertension using a dosage of nearly 2 g of EPA/day and nearly 3 g of DHA/day over 2 weeks. In patients with HLP, i.e. higher initial levels of serum triglycerides and cholesterol, even a lower dose (nearly 1 g of EPA/day and nearly 2 g of DHA/day) was effective. Since the most pronounced effects were seen in subjects with the highest initial values, the question arises of whether the lowering of serum lipids and lipoproteins can then be maintained by long-term intake of a lower dose of ω3 fatty acids. Results from recent studies are encouraging [35, 64]. Although the concomitant increase of HDL cholesterol did not reach the level of significance in all studies, it suggests a beneficial influence of the mackerel diet on a lipid constellation, which is generally accepted as atherogenic. The possible mechanisms involved have been discussed elsewhere [4, 20]. In short, it can be assumed that a reduced fatty acid synthesis [65] and a low activity of lipogenic enzymes [66] in liver cause a blunted hepatic VLDL formation and secretion. In the plasma, VLDL rapidly lose their triglycerides and are converted into LDL, which, accordingly, decrease likewise. (The decrease of LDL after fish diets described is dissimilar to several recent reports indicating an increase of LDL by fish oil supplements [for a review, see ref. 37].) This is in agreement with clinical observations that in the triglycerides of morphologically fat-free liver the percentage of EPA is high, becoming nearly 10 times lower in hepatic steatosis, when the triglyceride level is high [67]. This observation has led to the speculation that dietary intake of ω3 fatty acids may have a beneficial effect in patients with liver steatosis. In addition, the decrease of free fatty acids during a standardized glucose tolerance test after the mackerel diet (at least in patients with HLP) suggests a reduced peripheral lipolysis [68, 69] and, consequently, a lack of substrate for hepatic triglyceride synthesis.

This might be consistent with a significant depression of plasma noradrenaline (study 1), although this decrease could not be found in a psychophysiological stress test (study 2), probably due to methodological reasons (mild stressors, inadequate timing of blood sampling).

Possibly, the lipid-lowering effect of canned mackerel is of a similar magnitude as that obtained with fish oil supplements [31, 35, 36].

In patients with HLP, apolipoproteins AI and B remained unchanged after the fish diets. This finding differs from recent data, demonstrating a decrease of apolipoprotein B after fish oil supplement [31] and could be due to methodological differences (fish oil versus canned fish). On the other hand, the decrease of apolipoproteins CII and CIII is in agreement with the decline of apolipoprotein CIII found in a recent study irrespective of the phenotype of the HLP [31]. The unchanged ratio of apolipoprotein CII and CIII after the mackerel diet suggests that lipoprotein lipase is not significantly influenced, in agreement with reports of unaffected postheparin lipolytic activity in healthy subjects [4, 20, 70] after fish diet or fish oil supplements. Despite the unchanged lipolytic activity, an increased susceptibility to lipolysis of chylomicrons containing ω3 PUFA resulting in reduced postprandial lipoprotein levels has been suggested [4, 70]. This might be of clinical importance, considering the fact that the human body is in a postprandial state for many hours of the day and it has been hypothesized that atherosclerosis is a postprandial phenomenon [71].

The blood-pressure-lowering effect of canned mackerel was consistent in all 4 studies. In patients with HLP, in whom the range of the blood pressure values was wide enough to allow a subdivision of the patients into systolic blood pressure groups (equal and above 160 mm Hg or below), the higher blood pressure was more effectively decreased [1]. These results probably have a similar basis to the finding of the most pronounced effect of fish supplements on the highest serum lipid levels according to Wilder's law of initial value. A dose-response relationship between ω3 PUFA and blood pressure reduction has recently been described in patients with mild hypertension [64]. It seems encouraging that elevated blood pressure from mildly hypertensive subjects even declined while they ingested a relatively low dose of ω3 fatty acids (3 cans/week of mackerel, equivalent to 3.3 g of EPA/week, and 4.2 g of DHA/week, corresponding to 0.5 g of EPA/day and 0.6 g of DHA/day). This amount could be recommended for a long-term low-dose fish consumption from a primary prevention standpoint. In this context, it appears an interesting phenomenon that abnormally elevated values (of blood pressure) could be readily normalized, whereas lipid levels within the normal range were not influenced by the relatively low dose of ω3 fatty acids in the same patients [72]. Similar data from long-term studies in patients with HLP are not yet available. However, it seems reliable for the treatment of risk factors to decrease preferably those values which are out of the normal range.

The mechanisms of the blood-pressure-lowering effect remain uncertain. It can be speculated that changes in lipid composition and fluidity of cell membranes, changes in receptor sites of vasoactive hormones or neural transmitters and direct effects of prostaglandins of the 3-series on either the vessel wall [73, 74] or transmitter release [75, 76] are involved. This could result from the in vivo formation of prostaglandin I_3 after a cod liver oil or mackerel diet in man [58]. However, it cannot be excluded that an additional increase in the formation of prostaglandin I_2 after a mackerel diet [58] might be relevant [57]. Moreover, effects of EPA independent of the eicosanoid formation were postulated [77]. This has been reviewed recently [78]. A higher level of TxB_2, the metabolite of TxA_2, in plasma and urine from patients with essential hypertension as compared to normotensive subjects has been described [79, 80], indicating that it could be important for the pathogenesis of essential hypertension. This was not confirmed by a recent study [43] suggesting that metabolites of prostaglandins and thromboxanes are not different in normotensive and hypertensive subjects. In our studies the basal level of TxB_2 did not correlate with individual blood pressure. Since the increase of TxB_2 during the stress test (study 2) failed to occur after both dietary periods, it can be suggested that dietary intake of ω3 PUFA might preserve the organism against stress-induced alterations. This can be an interesting new, but widely unknown, indication of dietary ω3 fatty acids. In another trial (study 4), a mackerel diet, providing an amount of 2.2 g/day of EPA and 2.8 g/day of DHA, depressed thromboxane formation by 50% in hypertensive subjects, which is in agreement with a recent long-term study in volunteers [81]. The data appear plausible, since TxA_2 is known as one of the most potent vasoconstrictive substances. Its decrease might, therefore, be involved in the blood pressure lowering in hypertensive subjects.

Apart from many uncertainties, it can be concluded that the dietary intake of ω3 fatty acids is an important contribution within a broad spectrum of dietary modifications to treat mild hypertension and HLP. The preparation of fish meals might be unacceptable for some people under eating habits (including fast foods) in industrialized countries [82], so we have favored a diet supplemented with canned fish rich in ω3 PUFA. The preference of fish dishes does not exclude the recommendation of encapsulated fish oil for further increase of the ω3 PUFA intake or for subjects who cannot tolerate or who refuse fish consumption for various reasons. To our practical experience the combination of both fish diet and intake of fish oil capsules are readily accepted by most of our patients. A potential advantage is the fact that several risk factors of atherosclerosis can be benefitted simultaneously by ω3 PUFA.

Conclusion

The review of the literature leads us to conclude that LA-rich diets decrease total and LDL cholesterol and ω3 fatty acids of different degree of unsaturation and chain lengths (LNA, EPA and DHA), in addition, lower serum triglycerides in normal, hypertensive and hyperlipemic subjects during short-term fish diets. The decrease of free fatty acids after a mackerel diet might suggest that eicosanoids of the 3-series derived from EPA may be involved in a depression of peripheral lipolysis, which contributes to the decrease of serum triglycerides via blunted VLDL synthesis and secretion from the liver.

From the data presented, it appears that with respect to their lipid-lowering effect LNA- and EPA-rich diets are similar. Their common feature, the ω3 position of the double bonds, could be important for this mode of action. This is different from the blood-pressure-lowering effect, which is most pronounced during diets rich in long-chain ω3 fatty acids. Therefore, it might be speculated that for the triglyceride-lowering potency the ω3 position of the double bonds or the degree of unsaturation, and for the blood pressure-lowering effect the chain length (C_{20} of the eicosanoid precursors), are the determining chemical components of ω3 PUFA. To test this hypothesis, further intraindividual comparative studies are necessary.

References

1   Singer P, Berger I, Wirth M, Gödicke W, Jaeger W, Voigt S: Slow desaturation and elongation of linoleic and α-linolenic acids as a rationale of eicosapentaenoic acid-rich diet to lower blood pressure and serum lipids in normal, hypertensive and hyperlipemic subjects. Prostaglandins Leukotrienes Med 1986;24:173–193.

2   Singer P, Jaeger W, Berger I, Barleben H, Wirth M, Richter-Heinrich E, Voigt S, Gödicke W: Effects of dietary oleic, linoleic and α-linolenic acids on blood pressure, serum lipids, lipoproteins and the formation of eicosanoid precursors in patients with mild hypertension. J Hum Hypertens, 1990;4:227–233.

3   Harris WS, Connor WE, McMurry MP: The comparative reduction of the plasma lipids and lipoproteins by dietary polyunsaturated fats: Salmon oil versus vegetable oils. Metabolism 1983;32:179–184.

4   Goodnight SH, Harris WS, Connor WE, Illingworth DR: Polyunsaturated fatty acids, hyperlipidemia and thrombosis, Arteriosclerosis 1982;2:87–113.

5   Iacono JM, Dougherty RM, Puska P: Reduction of blood pressure associated with dietary polyunsaturated fat. Hypertension 1982;4(suppl III):34–42.

6   Rao RH, Rao UB, Srikantia SG: Effect of polyunsaturate-rich vegetable oils on blood pressure in essential hypertension. Clin Exp Hypertens 1981;3:27–38.

7   Comberg HU, Heyden S, Hames CG: Hypertensive effect of dietary prostaglandin precursor in hypertensive man. Prostaglandins 1978;15:193–197.

8   Vergroesen AJ, Fleischmann AI; Comberg HU, Heyden S, Hames CG: The influence of increased dietary linoleate on essential hypertension in man. Acta Biol Med Germ 1978;37:879–883.

9   Hoffmann P, Taube Ch, Heinroth-Hoffmann I, Fahr A, Beitz J, Förster W, Poleshuk WS, Markov ChM: Antihypertensive action of dietary polyunsaturated fatty acids in spontaneously hypertensive rats. Arch Int Pharmacodyn 1985;276:222–235.

10   Schoene NW, Reeves VB, Ferretti A: Effects of dietary linoleic acid on the biosynthesis of PGE_2 and PGF_2 in kidney medulla in spontaneously hypertensive rats. Adv Prostaglandin Thromboxane Res 1980;8:1791–1792.

11   Iacono JM, Marshall MW, Dougherty RM; Wheeler MA, Mackin JF, Canary JJ:

Reduction in blood pressure associated with high polyunsaturated fat diets that reduce blood cholesterol in man. Prev Med 1975;4:426–443.

12 Hoffmann P, Block H-U, Beitz J, Taube Ch, Förster W, Wortha P, Singer P, Naumann E, Heine H: Comparative study of the blood pressure effects of four different vegetable fats on young, spontaneously hypertensive rats. Lipids 1986;21:733–737.

13 Zöllner N, Adam O, Wolfram G: The influence of linoleic acid intake on the excretion of urinary prostaglandin metabolites. Res Exp Med 1979;175:149–153.

14 Dyerberg J, Bang HO, Aagard O: α-Linolenic acid and eicosapentaenoic acid. Lancet 1980;i:199.

15 Mest HJ, Beitz J, Heinroth I, Block HU, Förster W: The influence of linseed oil diet on fatty acid pattern in phospholipids and thromboxane formation in platelets in man. Klin Wochenschr 1983;61:187–191.

16 Singer P, Jaeger W, Voigt S, Thiel H: Defective desaturation and elongation of n–6 and n–3 fatty acids in hypertensive patients. Prostaglandins Leukotrienes Med 1984;15:159–165.

17 Horrobin DF: Loss of delta-6-desaturase activity as a key factor in aging. Med Hypotheses 1981;7:1211–1220.

18 Horrobin DF, Manku MS, Huang YS: Effects of essential fatty acids on prostaglandin biosynthesis. Biomed Biochim Acta 1984;43:S114–S120.

19 Horrobin DF: Essential fatty acids and the complications of diabetes mellitus. Wien Klin Wochenschr 1989;101:289–293.

20 Singer P, Jaeger W, Wirth M, Voigt S, Naumann E, Hajdu I, Gödicke W: Lipid and blood pressure-lowering effect of mackerel diet in man. Atherosclerosis 1983;49:99–108.

21 Singer P, Wirth M, Voigt S, Richter-Heinrich E, Gödicke W, Berger I, Naumann E, Listing J, Hartrodt W, Taube Ch: Blood pressure- and lipid-lowering effect of mackerel and herring diet in patients with mild essential hypertension. Atherosclerosis 1985;56:223–235.

22 Singer P, Wirth M, Berger I, Voigt S, Gerike U, Gödicke W, Köberle U, Heine H: Influence on serum lipids, lipoproteins and blood pressure of mackerel and herring diet in patients with type IV and V hyperlipoproteinemia. Atherosclerosis 1985;56:111–118.

23 Singer P, Wirth M, Gödicke W, Heine H: Blood pressure lowering effect of eicosapentaenoic acid-rich diet in normotensive, hypertensive and hyperlipemic subjects. Experientia 1985;41:462–464.

24 Royer ME, Ko K: A simplified semiautomated assay for plasma triglycerides. Anal Biochem 1969;29:405–411.

25 Singer P, Voigt S, Moritz V, Baumann R: The fatty acid pattern of triglycerides and FFA in serum of spontaneously hypertensive rats (SHR). Atherosclerosis 1979;33:227–238.

26 Singer P, Wirth M, Gerike U, Gödicke W, Moritz V: Age-dependent alterations of linoleic, arachidonic and eicosapentaenoic acids in renal cortex and medulla of spontaneously hypertensive rats. Prostaglandins 1984;27:375–390.

27 Lopes-Virella MF, Stone P, Ellis S, Colwell JA: Cholesterol determination in high-density lipoproteins separated by three different methods. Clin Chem 1977;23:882–884.

28   Friedewald WT, Levy RI, Fredrickson DS: Estimation of the concentration of low density lipoprotein cholesterol in plasma, without use of the preparative ultracentrifuge. Clin Chem 1972;18:499–502.

29   Puska P, Iacono JM, Nissinen A, Korhonen HJ, Vartiainen E, Pietinen P, Dougherty R, Leino U, Mutanen M, Moisio S: Controlled, randomised trial of the effect of dietary fat on blood pressure. Lancet 1983;i:1–5.

30   Singer P, Voigt S, Gödicke W: Inverse relationship between linoleic acid in serum and adipose tissue of patients with essential hypertension. Prostaglandins Leukotrienes Med 1982;9:603–613.

31   Phillipson BE, Rothrock DW, Connor WE, Harris WS, Illingworth DR: Reduction of plasma lipids, lipoproteins, and apoproteins by dietary fish oils in patients with hypertriglyceridemia. N Engl J Med 1985;312:1210–1216.

32   Mortensen JZ, Schmidt EB, Nielsen AH, Dyerberg J: The effect of n–6 and n–3 polyunsaturated fatty acids on haemostasis, blood lipids and blood pressure. Thromb Haemost 1983;50:543–546.

33   Dyerberg J, Mortensen JZ, Nielsen AH, Schmidt EB: n–3 polyunsaturated fatty acids and ischaemic heart disease. Lancet 1982;ii:614.

34   Von Lossonczy TO, Ruiter A, Bronsgeest-Schoute HC, van Gent CM, Hermus RJJ: The effect of a fish diet on serum lipids in healthy human subjects. Am J Clin Nutr 1978;31:1340–1346.

35   Saynor R, Verel D, Gillott T: The long-term effect of dietary supplementation with fish lipid concentrate on serum lipids, bleeding time, platelets and angina. Atherosclerosis 1984;50:3–10.

36   Nestel P, Connor WE, Reardon MF, Connor S, Wong S, Boston R: Suppression by diets rich in fish oil of very low density lipoprotein production in man. J Clin Invest 1984;74:82–89.

37   Harris WS: Fish oils and plasma lipid and lipoprotein metabolism in humans: A critical review. J Lipid Res 1989;30:785–807.

38   Dehmer GJ, Popma JJ, van den Berg EK, Eichhorn ED, Prewitt JB, Campbell WB, Jennings L, Willerson JT, Schmitz JM: Reduction in the rate of early restenosis after coronary angioplasty by a diet supplemented with n–3 fatty acids. N Engl J Med 1988;319:733–740.

39   Harris WS, Connor WE, McMurry MP: Reduction of plasma lipids and lipoproteins by dietary ω–3 fatty acids. Am J Clin Nutr 1980;33:928–935.

40   Sanders TB, Vickers M, Haines AP: Effect on blood lipids and haemostasis of a supplement of cod liver oil, rich in eicosapentaenoic and docosahexaenoic acids, in healthy young men. Clin Sci 1981;61:317–324.

41   Lorenz R, Spengler U, Fischer S, Duhm J, Weber PC: Platelet function, thromboxane formation and blood pressure control during supplementation of the Western diet with cod liver oil. Circulation 1983;67:504–511.

42   Norris PG, Jones CJH, Weston MJ: Effect of dietary supplementation with fish oil on systolic blood pressure in mild essential hypertension. Br Med J 1986;293:104–105.

43   Knapp HP, FitzGerald GA: The antihypertensive effects of fish oil: A controlled study of polyunsaturated fatty acid supplements in essential hypertension. N Engl J Med 1989;320:1037–1043.

44   Kato T, Wakui Y, Nagatsu T, Ohnishi T: An improved dual wavelength spectropho-
      tometric assay for dopamine-β-hydroxylase. Biochem Pharmacol 1978;27:829–
      831.

45   Da Prada M, Zürcher G: Simultaneous radioenzymatic determination of plasma
      and tissue adrenaline, noradrenaline and dopamine within the femtomole range.
      Life Sci 1976;19:1161–1174.

46   Thybusch D: Enzymatische Mikrobestimmung der Blutglukose mit dem Fermo-
      gnost-Blutzucker-Testbesteck. Z Med Labortech 1971;12:249–254.

47   Duncombe W: The colorimetric micro-determination of nonesterified fatty acids in
      plasma. Clin Chim Acta 1964;9:122–129.

48   Gottschling D, Ziegler M, Wilke W, Michael R: Radioimmunoassay von Plasmain-
      sulin – Methodenkritische Untersuchungen. Radiobiol Radiother 1974;15:91–
      102.

49   Richter-Heinrich E, Läuter J: A psychophysiological test as diagnostic tool with
      essential hypertensives. Psychother Psychosom 1969;17:153–168.

50   Taube C, Höhler H, Lorenz S, Förster W: The role of TxA$_2$ in hypertension. Biomed
      Biochim Acta 1984;43:S208–S211.

51   Fredrickson DS, Levy RI, Lees RS: Fat transport in lipoproteins – An integrated
      approach to mechanisms and disorders. N Engl J Med 1967;276:32–44, 94–103,
      148–156, 215–226, 273–281.

52   Laurell CB: Electroimmunoassay. Scand J Clin Invest 1972;172(suppl 124):21–37.

53   Gehrisch S, Jaross W: Isolierung und immunologische Bestimmung von Apolipo-
      protein C-II und C-III im menschlichen Serum. Z Med Lab Diagn 1985;26:157–
      165.

54   Patrono C, Ciabattoni G, Pinca E, Pugliese F, Castrucci G, de Salvo A, Satta MA,
      Peskar BA: Low dose aspirin and inhibition of thromboxane B$_2$ production in
      healthy subjects. Thromb Res 1980;17:317–327.

55   Deutsches Arzneibuch (DDR): Diagnostische Laboratoriumsmethoden, ed 7. Ber-
      lin, Akademie-Verlag, 1973.

56   von Euler US, Lishajko F: Improved technique for the fluorimetric estimation of
      catecholamines. Acta Physiol Scand 1961;51:348–356.

57   Singer P, Wirth M, Berger I, Heine H: Decrease of linoleic acid in serum lipids and
      increase of arachidonic acid in serum triglycerides after diets supplemented with
      n–3 fatty acids. Aktuel Ernähr 1989;14:264–268.

58   Fischer S, Weber PC: Prostaglandin I$_3$ is formed in vivo in man after dietary eico-
      sapentaenoic acid. Nature 1984;307:165–168.

59   Singer P, Gerhard U, Moritz V, Förster D, Berger I, Heine H: Different changes of
      n–6 and n–3 fatty acids in adipose tissue from spontaneously hypertensive (SHR)
      and normotensive rats after diets supplemented with linolenic or eicosapentaenoic
      acids. Prostaglandins Leukotrienes Med 1986;24:163–172.

60   Singer P, Berger I, Gerhard U, Wirth M, Moritz V, Förster D: Changes of n–6 and
      n–3 fatty acids in liver from spontaneously hypertensive (SHR) and normotensive
      rats after diets supplemented with α-linolenic or eicosapentaenoic acids. Prostaglan-
      dins Leukotrienes Med 1987;28:183–194.

61   Singer P, Wirth M, Kretschmer H, Berger I: Extreme decrease of linoleic acid in
      renal medulla from rats after a diet supplemented with cod liver oil. Prostaglandins
      Leukotrienes Essent Fatty Acids 1990;39:329–335.

62 Schoene NW, Fiore D: Effect of a diet containing fish oil on blood pressure in spontaneously hypertensive rats. Prog Lipid Res 1981;20:569–570.

63 Hornstra G, Christ-Hazelhof E, Haddeman E, ten Hoor F, Nugteren DH: Fish oil feeding lowers thromboxane and prostacyclin production by rat platelets and aorta and does not result in the formation of prostaglandin I_3. Prostaglandins 1981;21:727–738.

64 Bønaa KH, Bjerve KS, Straume B, Gram IT, Thelle D: Effect of eicosapentaenoic and docosahexaenoic acids on blood pressure in hypertension. N Engl J Med 1990;322:795–801.

65 Yang KT, Williams MA: Comparison of C_{18}-, C_{20}- and C_{22}-unsaturated fatty acids in reducing fatty acid synthesis in isolated rat hepatocytes. Biochim Biophys Acta 1978;531:133–140.

66 Iritani N, Inoguchi K, Endo M, Fukuda E, Moreta M: Identification of shellfish fatty acids and their effects on lipogenic enzymes. Biochim Biophys Acta 1980;618:378–382.

67 Singer P, Honigmann G, Schliack V: Decrease of eicosapentaenoic acid in fatty liver of diabetic subjects. Prostaglandins Med 1980;5:183–200.

68 Bergström S, Carlson LA, Orö L: Effect of prostaglandins on catecholamine-induced changes in the free fatty acids of plasma and in blood pressure in the dog. Acta Physiol Scand 1964;60:170–180.

69 Dalton C, Pope H, Martikes L: Prostaglandin inhibition of cyclic-AMP accumulation and rate of lipolysis in fat cells. Prostaglandins 1974;7:319–324.

70 Weintraub MS, Zechner R, Brown A, Eisenberg S, Breslow JL: Dietary polyunsaturated fats of the ω–6 and ω–3 series reduce postprandial lipoprotein levels. J Clin Invest 1988;82:1884–1893.

71 Zilversmit DB: Atherogenesis: A postprandial phenomenon. Circulation 1979;60:473–485.

72 Singer P, Berger I, Lück K, Taube Ch, Naumann E, Gödicke W: Long-term effect of mackerel diet on blood pressure, serum lipid and thromboxane formation in patients with mild essential hypertension. Atherosclerosis 1986;62:259–265.

73 Wendling MG, Du Charme DW: Cardiovascular effects of prostaglandin D_3 and D_2 in anaesthetized dogs. Prostaglandins 1981;22:235–243.

74 Hedqvist P: Basic mechanisms of prostaglandin action on autonomic neurotransmission. Annu Rev Pharmacol Toxicol 1977;17:259–279.

75 Hemker DP, Aiken JW: Effects of prostaglandin D_3 on nerve transmission in nictitating membrane of cats. Eur J Pharmacol 1980;67:155–158.

76 Dyerberg J, Jørgensen KA, Arnfred T: Human umbilical blood vessel converts all, cis-5,8,11,14,17 eicosapentaenoic acid to prostaglandin I_3. Prostaglandins 1981;22:857–862.

77 Pace-Asciak CR, Asotra S, Woodside M, Torchia J, Levine L: The antihypertensive action of 5,8,11,14,17-eicosapentaenoic acid ethyl ester (EPA-EE) may be direct effect without implicating the arachidonic acid cascade (abstract). Health Effects of Fish and Fish Oils, St. John's 1988.

78 Singer P: Blood pressure lowering effect of ω3 polyunsaturated fatty acids in clinical studies; in Simopoulos AP, Kifer RR Martin RE, Barlow SM (eds): Health Effects of ω3 Polyunsaturated Fatty Acids in Seafoods. World Rev Nutr Diet. Basel, Karger, 1991, vol 66, pp 329–348.

79 Hornych A, Safar M, Bariety J, Simon A: Thromboxane B_2 in borderline and essential hypertensive patients. Prostaglandins Leukotrienes Med 1983;10:145–155.

80 Chen LS, Ito T, Ogawa K, Shikano M, Satake T: Plasma concentrations of 6-keto-prostaglandin $F_{1\alpha}$, thromboxane B_2 and platelet aggregation in patients with essential hypertension. Jpn Heart J 1984;25:1001–1009.

81 von Schacky C, Fischer S, Weber PC: Long-term effect of dietary marine ω–3 fatty acids upon plasma and cellular lipids, platelet function, and eicosanoid formation in humans. J Clin Invest 1985;76:1626–1631.

82 Leaf A, Weber PC: Cardiovascular effects of n–3 fatty acids. N Engl J Med 1988; 318:549–557.

PD Dr. med. Peter Singer, Melibokusstr. 14, D-W–6140 Bensheim 3 (FRG)

Simopoulos AP (ed): Nutrients in the Control of Metabolic Diseases.
World Rev Nutr Diet. Basel, Karger, 1992, vol 69, pp 113–165

The Affluent Diet and Its Consequences: Saudi Arabia – A Case in Point

Ahmed A. Al-shoshan

Department of Nutrition, King Saud University, Ministry of Health, Riyadh, Saudi Aarabia

Contents

Introduction 113
Overnutrition and Global Trends 114
The Middle East: A Growing Concern 119
The Kingdom of Saudi Arabia 126
    Food Production, Imports and the Availability 126
    Dietary Habits, Consumption Pattern and Available Nutrients 129
    Trends in Chronic Diseases 142
Guidelines and Recommendations 153
    The Advocacy: Administrative and Political Support 153
    The Administrative Unit: The Infrastructure 154
    Intersectoral Food and Nutrition Planning Council 154
    National Food and Nutrition Policies 156
    Development of National Dietary Guidelines 156
    Mass Media and Public Awareness 156
    Nutritional Support Unit in Primary Health Care Centers, Clinics and
        Hospitals 157
    Role of the Food Industry 157
    Target-Oriented Education, Training, Extension and Research Activities . . 158
    The Ultimate: You, the Individual 159
Acknowledgments 160
References 161

Introduction

Malnutrition, like a coin, has two faces: undernutrition and overnutrition. Both have identical and equally grave consequences for mankind: increased susceptibility to diseases, reduced productivity and shortened life expectancy. Malnutrition, in both of its forms, has now become a medical scourge, an economic drain on national development and a major growing concern for global health [1].

It is not the aim of this article to review and dramatize the consequences of undernutrition; rather, it is to bring the alarming global trends of overnutrition to the attention of the public, media and concerned authorities. Similar to that of undernourishment, overnutrition, a gross imbalance between the caloric intake and expenditure, results in obesity which, in turn, can lead to major chronic killer diseases, such as diabetes, hypertension, cardiovascular diseases, kidney failure, certain types of cancer and the associated complications.

Hospitals, medications and industrialized health care delivery services can hardly be the answer for the consequences of malnutrition. Health authorities everywhere almost unanimously agree that the money spent to eradicate the etiology of a disease will pay greater economic returns than an extra billion spent for the development of a sophisticated medical apparatus, research purely designed to satisfy the scientific curiosity, or curative interventions administered to camouflage the symptoms of a disease [1, 2].

A new challenge now faces the developed affluent societies: how to combat the chronic health problems due to overnutrition and unique lifestyle associated with wealth, abundance and affluence. It is now a well-known fact that 7 out of the 10 leading causes of death are diet- and lifestyle-related maladies [3, 4]. This article briefly reviews the global trends of overnutrition, highlights the growing concerns in the Middle East, presents the stark realities of overnutrition, with facts and figures, for one of the affluent societies of the region, the Kingdom of Saudi Arabia, and recommends guidelines to the responsible authorities in order to partially reverse or, at least, to alleviate the grave consequences of overnutrition for generations to come.

Overnutrition and Global Trends

The affluent diet is a consumption pattern which flourishes where high-life and prosperity prevail. It is now sweeping the world with its lifestyle where per capita income is above that of optimum, such as industrialized western countries, those endowed with natural resources high in demand and urban elites with high purchasing power in the developing countries. This consumption pattern, in general, does appeal to the eye, pleases the taste buds and appears to be nutritionally satisfying. It is, however, rich in animal protein, fat, cholesterol, refined sugar, processed fruits and vegetables. Such a diet, although rich in nutrients, may very well be a life-threatening source of major health risk factors [1–3].

Epidemiological studies to date have clearly established a correlation between the dietary pattern and the prevalence of chronic killer diseases, such as obesity, hypertension, diabetes, cardiovascular disease and others [3]. The National Academy of Sciences of the USA reports that the role of diet is now documented in both the prevention and treatment of many chronic diseases and their related complications [3, 5, 6].

The affluent dietary pattern, with its prosperous sedentary life-style, may soon open new avenues to maladies and ailments that have never been recorded in the history of mankind. This new emerging trend, the so-called affluent diet, characterized with wealth, high standard of living, prosperity, high purchasing power, taste for rare commodities and a unique sedentary life-style, is now causing a global outbreak of health hazards which are sometimes referred to as 'diseases of civilization', or one may prefer to call them 'diseases of affluence' [1, 2].

During the last several decades or so, one could observe drastic changes in the world's food consumption pattern. In the industrialized western societies, such as the USA, up to 45% of the total caloric intake is composed of fat. The global average is over 40% in many western countries. The consumption of bulky foods, complex carbohydrates and fiber-rich foods has declined in favor of simple and refined sugar. Global per capita sugar consumption has also doubled, and the average person today consumes 44 lb of sugar per year. In some western countries, led by America, per capita refined sugar consumption exceeds over 100 lb per year [1].

As the affluent diet has spread around the world, so have the killer chronic diseases, such as obesity, cardiovascular diseases, hypertension, kidney failure and various types of cancer. A brief review of these chronic health hazards might shed some light on the grim outlook of their global trends [7].

Obesity is one of the most common public health problems of our time. It is the most prevalent form of malnutrition in the US [8, 9]. Obesity is a powerful predictor of virtually all cardiovascular end points in men and women. It is associated with elevated blood pressure, blood lipids and blood glucose, and is a major risk factor for diabetes, complications of pregnancy, osteoarthritis, certain types of cancer, infections and impaired psychosocial functions [5]. The National Center for Health Statistics reports that Americans, on the average, weigh more now than they did 10 years ago. Thirty-two percent of the men and 63% of the women in the US are 10% or more, and 18% of the men and 24% of the women weigh 20% or more above the ideal weight [5].

Traditionally restricted to the elite, obesity was regarded once as a status symbol. The Roman Senator's girth won him a great prestige among the mass of underfed plebeians; and Aga Khan's annual weighings were legendary among his people. In Nepal, obesity is a mark of distinction and a reducing diet is politically unacceptable. The double-chin epidemic, 'Doppelkinnepidemia', was widespread in postwar Germany. In the US today, 10–20% of all children and 35–50% of all middle-aged people are overweight. Lately, however, excessive fat has become the scourge of the lower socioeconomic class, and by western standard it is considered as social disdain. In our time, fewer and fewer jobs require physical work of any sort, and *Homo sapiens*, as pointed out by Eckholm and Record [1], has now become *Homo sedentarius*. Nevertheless, Hippocrates' dictum that the fat die sooner than the thin still remains an alarming fact today, as it did 2,000 years ago [1].

Coronary heart disease, once a rare affliction even among the old, is now the leading killer of the middle-aged in many countries. The affluent diet and sedentary life-style are the major contributing factors to this trend, not only in the industrialized rich countries, but also among the urban elites of the developing world [1, 2]. All cardiovascular diseases together, including coronary and other heart diseases, account for about one half of all deaths in the industrialized countries, and currently are the leading cause of death in the US adult population. Approximately 45 million Americans are affected by one or more forms of heart, blood vessel or cerebrovascular diseases, including hypertension, coronary heart disease and stroke [3, 5, 10]. Coronary heart disease alone accounts for 1 in every 3 deaths in the US, claiming annually more than 700,000 lives. In Japan and France, cerebrovascular disease or stroke takes even more lives than does coronary heart disease. Higher dietary intake of saturated fat and cholesterol are among the major factors. Doctors at the Bir Hospital in Kathmandu, Nepal, have noted that the annual number of heart attacks increased from 3 to 30 between the sixties and seventies, indicating that the affluent life-style in the capital city has been a major factor. In the Ivory Coast, the emergence of coronary heart disease among the more affluent class of Abidjan was reported by the health care officials in the seventies [1].

A WHO study showed that in 17 out of 22 countries studied in North and South America cardiovascular disease is now one of the 5 principal causes of death, and 9 of every 10 victims were male with an average age of 53 years. In 10 of these countries, heart disease is the No. 1 killer [11]. Public response to education programs designed to lower high blood pressure and to ensure the maintenance of its normal levels has been outstanding in the western world which is being led by the USA [5].

Hypertension, i.e. high blood pressure, is one of the most common illnesses of our time [12, 13]. It is associated with coronary heart disease, stroke, congestive heart failure and kidney diseases. In nearly all cases the actual cause of hypertension is unknown. The dietary factors, especially salt intake, are now believed to be the major causes in hypertension. Past and recent studies have firmly established a strong relationship between high salt consumption and high blood pressure in rats, strongly suggesting that high salt intake may contribute significantly to hypertension in man [14–16]. Obesity has been clearly established as a risk factor for both coronary heart disease and hypertension, and obese people who adopt special low-salt diets reduce their blood pressure long before they reduce their body weight [1]. Similar studies in the Bahamas, South Africa, Japan, US and Polynesia have all shown a relationship between high salt intake and hypertension [1]. In Japan, where northerners eat more salt than do the southerners, the greater incidence of hypertension in the north is apparently salt-related. On the average, Japanese have perhaps the world's highest salt intake rate which probably explains their exceptional susceptibility to stroke and hypertension [1].

Throughout the world, wherever there exists a pocket of affluence, so does the incidence of diabetes mellitus. In the developing parts of the world it appears to be mainly an urban disease, in affluent societies it afflicts both rural and urban alike. Once, in the early part of the present century, it was the 27th most common cause of death in the US; it has now captured the 5th place in the mid-seventies with all its side effects and complications, including retinopathy, nephropathy and neuropathy; its death toll follows the cardiovascular diseases and cancer. Again, the affluent diet plays an important role in this deadly disease all over the world. Overnutrition leading to obesity and predisposing to adult-onset diabetes appears to be associated with affluent diet and a sedentary life-style [1]. The majority of adult-onset diabetics is mainly due to overnutrition and obesity [17]. A person who is 20% overweight is more than twice as likely to develop diabetes as a person with normal weight. Reduction in food consumption, consuming less refined sugars, increasing complex carbohydrates and fibers in the diet, and maintaining a desirable weight help prevent this age-old chronic killer disease of overnutrition and sedentary life-style [18–20].

During the last several decades, environmental pollutants, radiation, chemicals, pesticides and food additives received considerable attention as carcinogens in the etiology of tumor formation [21, 22]. Throughout the seventies and eighties, although a great deal of research still needs to be done, more and more studies are now linking the diet and consumption patterns to the etiology of this major killer [23–27]. Growing evidence suggests that a high-fat diet does indeed contribute to the development of several important types of cancer, including those of the colon, rectum, breast and prostate [28, 29]. Not surprisingly, dietary influences are considered to promote cancers of the digestive system which include the mouth, throat, esophagus, stomach, colon and rectum. Diet has also been associated, throughout the metabolic processes, with some cancer sites outside the gastrointestinal tract, through hormonal imbalances, influenced by the abnormal dietary intake of certain nutrients, thus affecting a variety of organ sites [1]. Hutter [30] emphasized life-style, especially tobacco, and related 33% of all cancer death toll to diet, nutrition and the consumption patterns. Purtilo and Cohen [31] pointed out that a great variety of natural mutagens and carcinogens find their way into the food chain and, thus, to the modern affluent diet. Excessive fat and alcohol consumption has been studied in relation to many malignancies. A provocative hypothesis argues that a high-fiber diet can substantially reduce the likelihood of carcinoma of the colon [32].

Although still rare in many parts of the world, bowel (colorectal) cancer is one of the leading killers in the western world. The striking international differences suggest environmental and dietary, rather than genetic, factors. For instance, Japanese who migrate to the US are more prone to bowel cancer at the US rates, rather than at the low Japanese one, common in mainland Japan [33]. Breast cancer follows the same pattern as that of bowel cancer. It strikes more women in the western industrialized countries than in any other part of the world. Japanese women seldom develop breast cancer, and their chances of developing carcinoma increase sharply when they migrate to the West and adopt a new dietary pattern and life-style. Thus, both bowel and breast cancer seem to be related to western life-style and the affluent diet [1].

The role of the nitrosamines in the etiology of stomach cancer has been extensively studied [34]. For instance, a high incidence of stomach cancer in Japan appears to be associated with certain food items and cultural practices. Nitrate- and nitrite-treated pickled food, smoked fish and asbestos residues on talc-coated white rice might explain their role in carcinoma of the stomach lining. It is now well known that populations consuming large amounts of smoked fish have higher rates of stomach cancers [1]. Food additives, both intentional and unintentional, have also received considerable attention [35], The affluent societies, with their overrefined and processed food supply, are now being exposed to an ample source of food additives. These man-made chemicals, and their exact contributions to cancer rates and sites in the affluent societies, will someday be the major occupation of researchers worldwide [1].

Scientific investigations and observations, in several western countries, have now created a new necessity for the development of new national policies, strategies, and guidelines in order to deal with and respond to the consequences of affluent diet [36].

The Middle East: A Growing Concern

The consequences of the affluent diet are not restricted to the industrialized, wealthy nations. The health implications of the modern, sedentary life-style and its associated affluent diet are now increasingly being experienced and recognized among the economically better societies of the developing world. The middle East, by all means, is no exception [37].

Background information, covering land, demography and the socioeconomic indicators for the region, was presented elsewhere [38]. Although the lack of data and the reliability of those available are the major limiting factors, the information to date clearly indicates that the food production and imports have increased in the region over the last 2 decades due to immigration, urbanization and rapid population growth. Revenues, boosted by oil exports, have led to improvements of the socioeconomic indicators and higher gross domestic product (GDP). Affluence and its associated life-style have even spread to neighboring countries through labor migrations. Higher per caput income and population growth (fig. 1) have naturally increased the demand for food production and imports, which, in turn, resulted in high caloric availability, consumption and decline in numbers of undernourished people [39].

Food production has expanded at an accelerating rate in the region since 1960 (fig. 1). Dietary energy supply (DES), expressed as kilocalories

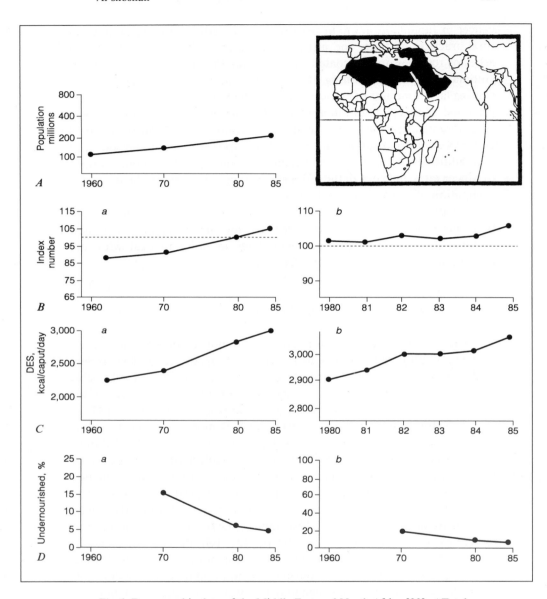

Fig. 1. Demographic data of the Middle East and North Africa [39]. *A* Total population: 1960–1985 (log scale). *B* Index numbers of per caput food production (1979/81 = 100). *a* 1960–1985: 3-year averages. *b* 1980–1985: annual. *C* DES. *a* 1960–1985; 3-year averages. *b* 1980–1985: annual. *D* Undernourished populations (DES < 1.2 BMR). *a* Percentage. *b* Numbers (millions).

per caput per day, the amount of food available to, not necessarily consumed by, household, due to imports, and ever-increasing food production showed a sharp increase (fig. 1). One can identify 3 groups of countries in the region. The group with the highest income (GDP/caput greater than $2,000), including Cyprus, Kuwait, Libya, Kingdom of Saudi Arabia and United Arab Emirates, had a DES estimated at more than 3,000 kcal/caput/day in 1979–1981. An intermediate-income group (GDP/caput of $1,000–2,000), with Algeria, Egypt, Iraq, Lebanon, Jordan, Morocco, Syria, Tunisia and Turkey, had a DES from 2,600 to 3,200 kcal/caput/day for the same period. The last group, with 2 low-income countries (GDP/caput lower than $1,000), the Yemes, had a DES of less than 2,300 kcal/caput/day [39]. Data from other sources are similar, or in complete agreement with those of the United Nations. Although the availability of energy supplies/calories does not necessarily reflect the amount consumed, they surely indicate the trends for the entire region [37, 38].

For the wealthier countries of the region, caloric availability increased at a rate approximately similar to that in other developing countries until the early seventies when economic prosperity accelerated with the oil boom. Since the mid-seventies, the rate of increase in caloric availability for these wealthy countries of the region, especially the Kingdom of Saudi Arabia, has been very fast, and by the early eighties (1981–1983) it far exceeded that of other countries, both developed or developing. The caloric availability for wealthier countries of the region is fast approaching the availability in the developed countries (fig. 2). If such a trend continues, by the mid-nineties the caloric availability will have exceeded that of the developed countries [37]. The prevalence of undernutrition, or marginal access to food, in the region is estimated to have fallen from 15 to only 6% between 1969–1971 and 1979–1981, and continued to decline, somewhat slowly, throughout the eighties (fig. 1). Even with the population growth, the numbers of undernourished people in the region has fallen from an estimated figure of 20 million in the early seventies to 10 million or lower in the early eighties (fig. 1) [39].

The increased GDP, wealth, prosperity and income distribution in the region have resulted in unique changes in life-style and associated consumption patterns [38]. There has been a drastic change in food consumption patterns and dietary habits as a result of the high income and associated prosperity. Musaiger [38] described the seventies, the so-called oil boom period, as the 'golden decade' for the Gulf region, and pointed out the invasion of western civilization in every household in the region. The

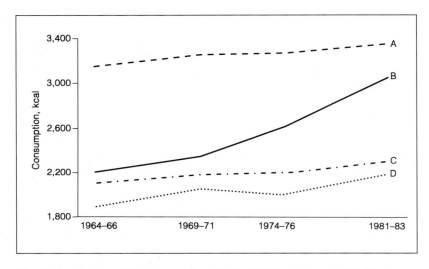

Fig. 2. Changes in calorie consumption (1964–1983) in the eastern Mediterranean (EM) region. A = Developed nations; B = wealthier nations of the EM region; C = developing nations; D = poorer nations of the EM region.

traditional diet, which consists of dates, milk, rice, bread and fish, has changed to a more diversified diet. Red meat is consumed more frequently than fish or poultry, and lamb and mutton are preferred over beef. More roots and tubers, fruits and vegetables, sugars and animal products are being consumed. Consumption of maize and barley has declined in many countries of the region, often accompanied by increased intake of wheat and rice. There has been a sharp increase in fat consumption mostly from imported vegetable oils. Poultry production has become a growing industry with the consumption of young broilers replacing traditional meats, such as sheep and goat. Average per caput meat consumption, which was around 10–12 kg per year in most countries 20 years ago, is now around 30 kg in many countries, and even exceeds 50 kg in some of the richest [38]. Rice is still the dominating staple cereal, and it is consumed daily. Wheat is consumed mainly as bread or macaroni. Tea is the most popular drink, sweetened, with or without milk. Canned and processed foods are widely available on the market and play an important role in the daily diet. The availability of more than 1,900 different kinds of processed foods from 38 countries in Bahrain alone was reported, and the figure could easily be doubled in larger countries, such as Kuwait and the Kingdom of Saudi Arabia [38].

Food adulteration, use of unsafe additives, mislabeling and improper packaging are frequently noticed in the Gulf region. It is generally believed that the people in the Gulf area are consuming processed foods with unsafe additives, coloring agents and carcinogens, and this has been creating a major health concern and awareness in the mind of the general public. Musaiger [38] emphasized both the positive and negative consequences of the rapid socioeconomic progress in the region. Farrag [40] summarized other sociopsychological changes, including decline in breast-feeding and early introduction of bottle feeding throughout the golden decade. A more recent study, however, investigating the infant feeding patterns and weaning practices in Kuwait, revealed some gratifying outlook in regard to breast-feeding patterns in the region [41]. The investigation, including 2,994 mothers of children less than 3 years of age, showed that 60.6% of the infants were being breast-fed, 13.6% were on the bottle and 25.8% received both feedings. It is interesting to note that older and illiterate mothers are more likely to breast-feed their infants for a longer period, and mothers from high-income families are less likely to practice breast-feeding [41].

According to a WHO report [37], the majority of calories available are contributed by the consumption of fats. Protein availability, expressed as grams per caput per day, not necessarily the amount consumed, also shows a steady increase in the region. The data clearly indicate a trend of increasing consumption of animal protein, especially red meats, eggs, milk and milk products. While the shortage of protein is clearly not a problem in the region, the interesting trend is the type of protein consumed. One may speculate, however, that the higher consumption of animal proteins could lead to a higher incidence of cardiovascular diseases in the area. While most of the western societies are now realizing that the substitution of carbohydrates for fats is an important step for the prevention of cardiovascular diseases, the trend among the wealthy nations of the region, unfortunately, is in the opposite direction [37].

Refined wheat products have almost doubled in the last 10 years or so in Saudi Arabia alone, and simultaneously sorghum consumption went down way below to what it was in 1976. Sugar consumption, known to be associated with elevated blood lipids and cariogenesis, has also increased for the countries in the region. Similarly, high salt intake has also found its way through the overrefined and processed food products and dietary patterns which are known to be associated with high blood pressure [37]. Although the affluence and associated dietary changes in the region have contributed a great deal to the general improvement of optimum nutrition, the health problems of dietary origin and the consequences of sedentary life-style and overnutrition have now become a growing concern in the Middle East [37, 38].

Obesity, as a common ground for all major chronic degenerative diseases, has now been recognized as a major risk factor, and its health implications are well established [4, 6, 42]. Although there have been no valid and well-executed studies on the prevalence of obesity in the region, it is highly believed that it is becoming one of the most important public health problems in the eastern Mediterranean region, predominantly among middle-aged adults (childhood obesity, most alarmingly, is also on the rise) [38]. The data, based on limited national surveys from Egypt and Kuwait, clearly signal the prevalence of adult obesity predominantly among females, 50% or more, in the region [37]. In a Kuwait community, where 9,000 males and 9,500 females were the subjects it was found that the prevalence of obesity increased with age. A rapid rate of increase was especially noticeable between adolescence and 40 years of age, and for males a peak was observed between the ages of 29 and 40, an obesity pattern similar to that of western societies [37]. Other small-scale studies were also conducted among certain groups in the region. Sedentary lifestyle and excessive caloric intake were the common ground in all these surveys [38]. Recently, Al-Awaidi and Amine [43] studied the factors affecting the prevalence of obesity among adult females in Kuwait. Observing a multistage stratified sample of over 3,000 females, the authors concluded that the prevalence of obesity was 42%, while underweight represented only 2.4% of the sample studied. Among the factors influencing the prevalence of obesity in the region were unemployment, illiteracy of both spouses, number of offspring and age of the subject. Family income, however, was inversely related to the prevalence of obesity. The lower the income the higher the incidence of obesity. Childhood obesity is also on the rise in the region. Considering the fact that most obese adults were once obese children, then the significance of this alarming trend deserves immediate attention [37, 38, 42].

In spite of the fact that the surveys conducted in the region were restricted to small sample sizes and can hardly be representative of the population in question, the available data indicate a high prevalence of diabetes mellitus comparable to that in the developed world [37]. The high incidence of diabetes and its heavy burden on the health care services in the region has also been extensively reviewed by Musaiger [38]. The author identified the factors which contribute to the high incidence of diabetes in the Gulf countries and provided a list of recommendations for its alleviation [38].

In the region, the only reliable information concerning cardiovascular diseases is in the form of hospital mortality data. According to an earlier review [37], nearly all the countries in the region show a high proportion of mortality from cardiovascular diseases. Musaiger [38] also stated that the cardiovascular diseases are one of the major causes of mortality among adults, 40 years and older, in the Gulf region. He pointed out the realities with the following statement: 'Affluence, associated dietary habits, hypertension, obesity and diabetes, as well as stress of modern life-style, smoking and alcoholism seem to be largely responsible for the increased morbidity and mortality from this major killer disease'. Among all these factors, the author singled out the affluent diet as the most important factor for the prevalence in the region [38]

A situation analysis carried out by the WHO [37] confirmed the findings by citing the rate of increase in Kuwait over the last 10 years. According to the report, cardiovascular diseases have increased, as sole cause of death, in absolute numbers by 10% over a 10-year period or by about 30% over the mortality rate in 1977 [37]. As a risk factor, cigarette smoking and alcohol consumption were also reported to be increased in the region. In Bahrain, imports of tobacco products increased from 857,000 kg in 1980 to 1,131,000 kg in 1984, an increase of 32%. In terms of dollar value, it represents $8.8 million and $14 million, respectively. Similar trends were also observed in other Gulf countries. In Saudi Arabia, for instance, values jumped from $165 million in 1982 and reached $243 million in 1983, an increase of 47%. A jump of 82% was recorded in the early eighties for the United Arab Emirates. High alcohol consumption, a recognized risk factor in cardiovascular diseases, has also shown a gradual increase in certain parts of the region where tolerated and permitted. The amount of alcoholic drinks consumed in Bahrain has increased from 7.4 million kg in 1979 to 10.3 million kg in 1982 [38].

High blood pressure, i.e. hypertension, is a chronic medical problem to which a significant portion of cardiovascular diseases and a large number of end-stage renal diseases, both acute and chronic, can be attributed [37]. The only trend information for the region, which requires careful interpretation, is the mortality data from hypertension. Available data from the countries of the region indicate an increasing trend. The prevalence of hypertension in Kuwait is around 16.1% in women and 22.6% in men. Data from Egypt confirm the fact that the prevalence of hypertension increases with age [37]. Sodium content was found to be very high in most dishes due to added salt in addition to the ample use of spices, especially cumin, coriander leaves and cloves. These spices are reported to contain higher amounts of sodium and, thus, more attention should be paid to local dishes, since hypertension is a common health problem in the Gulf area. It was also confirmed that most of the various types of breads consumed in Bahrain were higher in sodium content due to the high salinity of the water used in preparation, in addition to the added salt [38].

In all countries of the region, as reported by the WHO [37], cancer rates seem to be on the rise. Data on cancers, as reported, come mainly from the mortality data. A trend of increasing prevalence is evident for breast cancer in Egypt and Kuwait, and for cancers of the digestive organs in Cyprus and Egypt. Trends appear to follow the pattern of those industrialized nations of the west. A cautious interpretation, however, must be taken into consideration [37].

The two most prevalent oral diseases in the Gulf and the surrounding countries are cariogenesis and periodontal diseases. The changes in dietary habits and consumption patterns have significantly contributed to the prevalence of cariogenesis. Sugar consumption has almost doubled between the years of 1975–1980. The fluoride content of the drinking water and the large consumption of bottled water, especially among the affluent people, are also among the contributing factors in the prevalence of cariogenesis. Musaiger [38] stressed the lack of oral hygiene, leading to gingivitis and periodontal diseases, in the Gulf countries and attributed it to the lack of national policies and programs.

The Kingdom of Saudi Arabia

Food Production, Imports and the Availability

In order to achieve the objectives of 'food self-sufficiency', reduce the volume of food imports and increase the agricultural productivity, the Ministry of Agriculture, through the channel of the Saudi Arabian Agricultural Bank and other agencies, embarked on very ambitious agricultural investment programs in the late seventies. The Saudi Government has made food self-sufficiency one of its utmost priorities and the progress

Table 1. Total supply of food choices (in thousand of tons) in Saudi Arabia from 1974 to 1986 [44]

Food choices	1974–1976	1977–1979	1980–1982	1983–1986	1974–1986, %
Cereals	984.6	1,482.1	1,972.5	2,350.0	138.7
Potatoes	16.7	38.1	74.9	83.9	402.4
Sugars	131.4	164.2	378.4	347.4	164.4
Meat	2,679.9	2,346.1	2,695.0	338.9	−87.4
Chicken	57.4	147.4	263.5	350.1	509.9
Fish	24.3	37.7	70.0	88.4	263.8
Dairy	264.3	412.3	437.1	489.3	85.1
Eggs	19.7	41.1	66.6	122.5	471.1
Fat/oils	27.2	87.0	149.4	194.4	614.7
Vegetables	496.5	645.8	864.5	1,273.8	156.6
Fruits	814.2	1,267.6	1,639.8	1,921.6	136.0
Pulses	19.9	38.5	65.2	87.5	339.7
Nuts	19.8	35.0	54.5	55.0	177.9

achieved to date, within a few years, has been unique and unprecedented anywhere around the world. Next to oil, agricultural industry is now the most important and impressive activity in the Kingdom. The country is witnessing an unparalleled full-scale farming boom, with agriculture's contribution to the Kingdom's GDP estimated to be on the rise since the early eighties [44, 45].

These and other advances in Saudi agriculture have received international attention. The Ministry of Agriculture was awarded a certificate of merit by the Food and Agriculture Organization of the United Nations in recognition of its work in helping Saudi Arabia to become self-sufficient in wheat production and other food commodities [44, 45]. The supply of food choices available to the consumer in the Kingdom during the period of 1974–1986 is presented in table 1. Accordingly, table 2 reflects the major food groups, in thousands of tons, during the same period. From the mid-seventies to the mid-eighties, egg production jumped from 204 million to 1.2 billion. As a result, the Ministry of Agriculture announced that the Kingdom was producing enough eggs not only to meet its own needs, but also to begin exports to other countries in the region. Self-sufficiency in dairy products has also been achieved since the mid-eighties, and more than 20 new dairy farms, since the early eighties, gave the country the

Table 2. Total supply of food groups (in thousand of tons) in Saudi Arabia from 1974 to 1986 [44]

Food groups	1974–1976	1977–1979	1980–1982	1983–1986
Starch and sugars	1,132	1,685	2,425	2,781
Meat	2,761	2,531	3,028	777
Fruits and vegetables	1,260	1,913	2,504	3,195
Dairy and eggs	284	453	503	601
Fat and oil	27	87	149	194

largest number of highly efficient dairy farms in the Middle East. The Kingdom's average milk yield, almost 7,000 liters per cow per year, is one of the best and most impressive in the world. Local poultry production rose by almost 60% in 1983 to about 145,000 t. Record production levels have also been achieved in fisheries with a production capacity of over 300,000 t per year. Livestock industry, with all feasible and approved projects, will enable the Kingdom to meet its rising demand for meat products by the nineties.

The most striking accomplishment in Saudi agriculture throughout the eighties has been the enormous production of cereal grains, particularly wheat. The production has increased from 26,000 t in the late sixties to over 26 million tons in the mid-eighties. Sales and donations of wheat abroad now exceed 1 million tons per year [44]. With the wheat production as the centerpiece of the agricultural sector, Saudi Arabia has moved from being a major importer to a net exporter of wheat in only 4 years. The only other crop which provides an exportable surplus is dates. Its production has increased from 240,000 to 475,000 t at an average annual rate of 4.9%, during the same period.

The agricultural sector in Saudi Arabia has enormous growth potential, and each year an increasing percentage of the country's food needs has been met by local production. With care and continued attention, agriculture in Saudi Arabia can be one of the world's greatest success stories. The agricultural sector, however, is small, about 5% of the GDP and 8% of the total labor force, but expanding rapidly, averaging over 8% per year during the eighties even as the overall GDP declined rapidly [46, 47]. About 75% of the food supply, however, is still imported. Almost all of Saudi requirements for cooking oil, fat, fresh fruits and vegetables, rice and sugars are imported [45]. Its imports have annually averaged 5 billion dollars during the mid-eighties. The US supplies about a seventh of the total food imports [45, 47]. In this drive for agricultural self-sufficiency, the government has employed modern agricultural policy tools with an impressive result. In spite of all these unparalleled achievements, however, the government also inherited some of modern agriculture's most persistent problems; among the most pressing ones are (1) surpluses of wheat, dates and eggs, (2) growing storage problems for grains and cereals, (3) an increasing financial drain on the national budget, (4) an influencial agricultural lobby and (5) a paucity of politically acceptable solutions. These problems, although feasible resolutions, have been exacerbated by stubbornly declining oil revenues throughout the eighties. With over 75% of its food supply imported, the government's political vulnerability, and thus food security, has now become the policy priority for the administration to tackle for the years to come. In spite of all these delicate food and agricultural policies, dependency on imported food commodities has diminished only slightly [47–49].

Dietary Habits, Consumption Pattern and Available Nutrients

These unparalleled social and economic progresses and developments in the region, within a decade or so, impacted all aspects of life in the Kingdom; the consumption patterns, dietary habits and associated lifestyle, naturally, were no exception.

As an important part of the Kingdom's development programs, the Multipurpose Household Survey (MPHS), which was carried out by the Central Department of Statistics, Ministry of Finance and National Economy, during the summer of 1982, brought out an interesting profile in regard to Saudi dietary habits and consumption patterns. Previously collected nutrition data, from April to October 1978, were utilized as supplement in this survey [50]. The compiled report provides data on nutrition in the Kingdom of Saudi Arabia which reflect the types of foods and drinks consumed and the number of meals eaten daily by the nonmigratory population. The information is based on 24-hour recall questionnaires, and the figures obtained reflect the servings per day which are based on a maximum of 4 per day for any specific food, regardless of the size of servings at each sitting. Therefore, 2 cups of tea for breakfast are counted as one serving only, and 5 cups dispersed throughout the day between meals are also counted as only one serving. This concept of servings, rather than the quantitites of foods consumed, is used throughout this survey (MPHS)

Table 3. Most commonly chosen foods for all nationalities [50]

Rank	Food	Servings	
		total number	number per person
1	Tea	18,356,544	1.80
2	Onion	12,234,010	1.20
3	Tomato	11,542,594	1.13
4	Rolled white bread	10,932,956	1.07
5	Rice	8,976,450	0.88
6	Whole wheat	5,432,783	0.53
7	Yellow cheese	4.899,313	0.48
8	Lamb	4,747,097	0.47
9	Arabic coffee	4,519,332	0.44
10	Fresh milk	4,005,543	0.39
11	Egg	3,954,881	0.39
12	Chicken	3,451,121	0.34
13	Dates	3,311,006	0.33
14	Olive	3,244,732	0.32
15	Bean	3,120,006	0.31
16	Pepsi	2,946,664	0.29
17	Buttermilk	2,849,423	0.28
18	Orange	2,453,658	0.24
19	Dry milk	1,999,935	0.20
20	Watermelon	1,897,254	0.19
21	Cream	1,810,387	0.18
22	Potato	1,737,019	0.17
23	Camel fallow	1,733,779	0.17
24	Banana	1,522,481	0.15
25	Apple	1,514,524	0.15

because the types of foods eaten at different sittings are far more sensitive measures than the quantities consumed at a sitting for the evaluation of nutritional levels or adequacy. In addition, the communal pattern of eating, eating from one large plate, often makes it extremely difficult to determine the actual quantities of each food ingested by an individual, and 'an average serving' per person may reflect heavy consumption of the food or drink by one, and total abstinence by the other [50].

The most popular food or drink consumed by the population of Saudi Arabia during August 1982, excluding sugar and salt, was tea which was drunk over 18 million times during a 24-hour recall period for an average

Table 4. Most commonly chosen foods for Saudis only [50]

Rank	Food	Servings	
		total number	number per person
1	Tea	12,400,977	1.77
2	Onion	8,773,970	1.25
3	Tomato	8,115,852	1.16
4	Rice	6.584,462	0.94
5	Rolled white bread	6,224,712	0.89
6	Arabic coffee	4,061.391	0.58
7	Whole wheat bread	4,040,222	0.58
8	Lamb	3,490,167	0.50
9	Dates	3,130,096	0.45
10	Yellow cheese	3,116,079	0.44
11	Fresh milk	2,791,019	0.40
12	Egg	2,514,346	0.36
13	Buttermilk	2,406,409	0.34
14	Olive	2,129,305	0.30
15	Chicken	2,059,037	0.29

of 1.8 daily servings per person. The remainder of the 10 most popular foods eaten in Saudi Arabia, excluding seasoning, includes onions, tomatoes, rolled white bread, rice, whole wheat bread, yellow cheese, lamb, arabic coffee and fresh milk. Each of these were consumed at least 4 million times during the 24-hour survey period for a daily average of more than one third serving per person. These 10 foods accounted for approximately 57% of all the types of foods consumed during the 24-hour reference day. The leading 25 foods accounted for 77% of all food consumed. The types of foods included represent a relatively high level of essential nutrients. The most commonly chosen 25 foods for all nationalities are presented in table 3 and table 4 indicates the most commonly chosen foods by the Saudi Nationals [50].

Meal Frequency. According to the survey (MPHS), about 96% of the total population ate at least 3 meals during the survey day, and most of these also supplemented their meals with in-between drinks or snacks. This proportion increased to an average of over 98% eating at least 3 meals per day for persons 5 years and older. The survey also indicated little difference between the sexes or between Saudis and non-Saudis in the frequency of meals eaten. Within the 3 meals/day group, however, the Saudis were more likely than their non-Saudi counterparts to have between-meal drinks or snacks in addition to their regular meals. For infants the data indicate frequent breast- or formula-feeding or supplemented by regular meals. Thus, for example, 64% of those under 1 year of age were breast-fed and 51% of those under 4 years of age were formula-fed, whereas more than 29% under 1 and more than 5% aged 1–4 had no regular meals. The 4% of persons in all age groups who ate fewer than 3 meals per day showed various combinations of breakfast, lunch and dinner with or without snacks. There was also relatively little difference in the regularity of meals among the 4 marital status groups or among the several education-literacy groups, except possibly for those with disrupted marriages, divorced, separated or widowed, who were less likely to supplement 3 regular meals with snacks than the currently married or the never-married persons [50].

Diet Quality and Adequacy. 'Dietary quality' in Saudi Arabia utilizes the '7 basic food groups' as follows: (1) leafy green and yellow vegetables; (2) citrus fruits and tomatoes; (3) potatoes and other vegetables and fruits; (4) milk and milk products; (5) meat and meat substitutes; (6) bread and cereals, and (7) vitamin-enriched fats and oils, and a special group for beverages and sweets. A substantial proportion of persons in Saudi Arabia ate 1 or more servings daily in each of the 7 basic food groups considered essential for good health. Therefore, a high proportion in each of the 7 basic food groups implies a diversity in the Saudi diet rather than concentrations in any one or two of the basic groups. According to the survey, the Saudis had a more diverse daily diet among the 7 basic food groups than their non-Saudi counterparts in the Kingdom [50].

Diet quality, in this survey, utilizes the 7 basic food groups method. The central core of the method is that the total nutrient requirements may be subsumed under these 7 groups. To meet these requirements, food from each group should be consumed a recommended number of times each day. When the number of servings per day meet or exceed these minima, then the food intake for individual or for groups is considered to be adequate. The percent adequacy is the proportion of persons who meet adequacy levels for a given or all food groups. According to survey findings, with the exception of 2 food groups, yellow and green vegetables and milk and milk products, 80% and above of all Saudi males and females had, at least, met or exceeded the recommended daily minimum of 3 or more

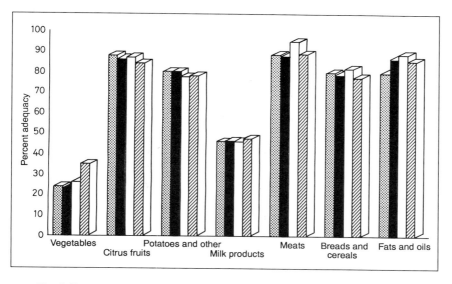

Fig. 3. Percent adequacy of foods eaten. ▦ = Saudi male; ■ = Saudi female; □ = non-Saudi male; ▨ = non-Saudi female.

servings of the other food groups. For the remaining 2 categories, the adequacy figures were low at 46% for both Saudi males and females having at least the recommended minimum of 2 daily servings of leafy green and yellow vegetables, and 24% of Saudi males and 23% of Saudi females having at least the minimum of 1 daily serving of milk and milk products (fig. 3). For both Saudi males and females, older persons had lower proportions meeting or exceeding the recommended minimum daily servings of the 7 basic food groups than did those in the young or middle age groups. The very young infants were also low in some categories because much of their nourishment came from formula- or breast-feeding rather than from the regular foods of the basic 7 groups [50].

It is interesting to note that the percent adequacy of servings in each of the 7 basic food groups tended to increase with the level of education of Saudi males and females. The survey also indicated that for all 7 basic food groups, except the bread and cereal group, there was an increase for Saudis in the percent adequacy from rural to urban and up to metropolitan areas. For breads and cereals, metropolitan areas were higher in levels of intake than rural areas (fig. 4). The eastern region had the highest percent ade-

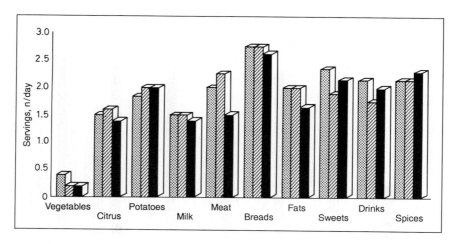

Fig. 4. Average servings per day by residence. ▦ = Metropolitan; ▨ = other urban, ■ = rural.

quacy of daily servings for Saudis in the 2 basic food groups of milk products and meats and meat substitutes, and shared the highest position with the central region in the group of potatoes and other fruits and vegetables (fig. 5). The central region was also highest in the citrus fruits, tomatoes and vitamin-fortified fats and oil groups. The western region was highest in bread and cereal groups, and lowest in yellow and leafy green vegetables. The southern region had the lowest daily levels of serving adequacy for Saudis in all food groups except bread and cereals. The northern region was the lowest for leafy green and yellow vegetables, and highest for bread and cereals [50].

Another approach is to measure average servings for the aggregated population, thus providing insights into the relative levels of intake of the 7 basic foods groups for the population as a whole, rather than to measure food intake adequacies for individuals only. If such approach is being utilized, the total population living in Saudi Arabia in August 1982 consumed: 1.7 daily servings of meat and meat substitute products as compared with the recommended 1.0 servings; 1.9 servings of potatoes or vegetables other than leafy green or yellow, or almost twice the recommended daily servings; 1.5 servings compared with 1.0 of citrus fruits or tomatoes; 1.8 servings as against 1.0 of fat and oils; 1.5 daily servings or slightly below the recommended 2.0 servings of milk and milk products, only 0.3

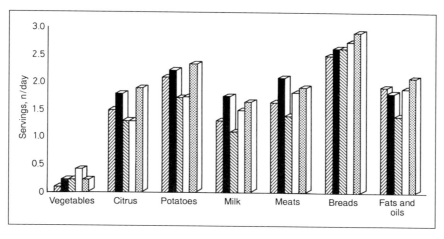

Fig. 5. Major foods by regions in Saudi Arabia. ▨ = North; ■ = east; ▧ = south; ☐ = west; ▦ = central.

servings or well below the recommended 1.0 serving of leafy green or yellow vegetables, and 2.6 servings as compared with the recommended 3.0 servings of bread and cereals. The bread and cereal intake in the Kingdom probably exceeds the recommended minimum because breads, rice and grain products are generally eaten in large quantities, and the type of bread is unique [50].

With the exception of infants and the aged, the middle-aged groups ate similar levels of food within each of the 7 food groups. Between the ages of 5 and 59 years, the variation in the average number of servings was only 0.1 or 0.2 of a serving in each of 7 basic food groups, and varied only at 0.4 of a serving in the remaining meat and meat substitute group (fig. 6). Literates consumed a greater average number of servings than illiterates in the basic food groups of citrus fruits, milk and milk products, meat and meat substitutes, and fat and oils, and were about the same in the remaining 3 groups. The overall outlook suggests that the literate and better-educated population either had more knowledge or higher purchasing power and resources to indulge in better diets than did the illiterate and less educated population. Slightly more than 1% of the population reported that they were on a special diet during the 24-hour recall survey. Of these, 18% were on a special diet because of a diabetic condition, 18% gave weight (obesity) as the reason for the diet, 12% hypertension, 11%

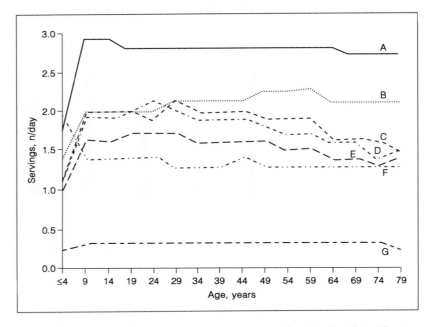

Fig. 6. Average servings per day of the major selected foods in Saudi Arabia. A = Bread and cereals; B = potatoes and others fruits; C = milk and milk product; D = meats, E = vegetables (yellos, green); F = citrus fruits; G = fats and oil.

reasons of allergies, 4% kidney and ulcers, 2% pregnancy and the remaining 35% cited unspecified personal reasons for a special diet [50].

Impressive agricultural productivity and a generous worldwide supply of imported food have all their impacts on the food consumption patterns and nutrient availability throughout the Kingdom. The trends for annual per capita consumption of food stuff and the nutrient availability for the period of 1974–1986 are presented in figures 7–14 [51].

The Kingdom's achievements of self-sufficiency and export in egg production in the mid-eighties has simultaneously accelerated its consumption, and within 10 years the consumption of eggs more than tripled. Per capita consumption of dairy products reached its peak during the late seventies and has started to decline slightly throughout the eighties. Availability of various soft drinks and other imported rare beverages may very well be the reason for the decline. Annual per caput consumption of total meat, including fish, poultry and red meat, has shown a steady increase through-

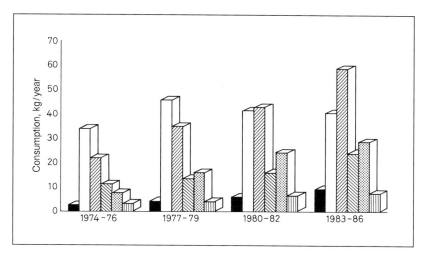

Fig. 7. Yearly per caput consumption of eggs (■), dairy products (□), total meat (▨), red meat (▧), poultry meat (▨) and fish (▥).

out the seventies and eighties. Affluence, high purchasing power and the availability of ample sources of raw and processed meat products in the market are the major contributing factors. A linear increase of total meat consumption in the eighties, from 22 to 60 kg/caput/year and above, confirms these observations (fig. 7) [51]. Per caput consumption of fats and oils as well as pulses have also shown a steady increase throughout the eighties. A decline in nut consumption, however, for some unknown reasons, possibly the emigration of foreign workers and changes in Saudi lifestyle, was recorded from the mid-eighties. A sharp increase in the late seventies and again a sharp decline in the mid-eighties in per caput consumption of sugars, from 16.1 to 35 kg/caput/year, and down to 28.1 kg/caput/year, might very well have been due to the high purchasing power and ample availability of various sugar products in the market, than to the decline in oil revenue, and thus purchasing power, and to the public awareness of its role in elevated blood lipid levels and cariogenesis, respectively. The annual consumption of fruits and vegetables showed a similar increase during the same period (fig. 8, 9) [51].

High consumption of cereals is the main feature of a Saudi diet (fig. 10). Wheat, rice and sorghum are the major staples. The success story of wheat production, its ever-increasing annual per caput consumption

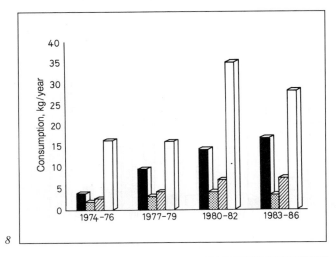

8

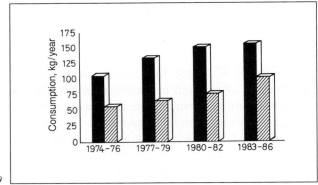

9

Fig. 8. Yearly per caput consumption of fats and oils (■), nuts (▒), pulses (▨) and sugar (□).

Fig. 9. Yearly per caput consumption of fruits (■) and vegetables (▨).

[10] and its popularity in Saudi dishes reflected itself as a decline in per caput consumption of sorghum. By the mid-eighties, its consumption declined to 3.2 from almost 15 kg/caput/year in the mid-seventies (fig. 11) [51]. Fats, both of animal and plant origin, showed a steady increase, jumping from 33.6 g/caput/day in the mid-seventies to 95 g/caput/day in the mid-eighties (fig. 12). Although a slight decline was observed in the consumption of plant protein, from 48.4 g/caput/day in the early eighties

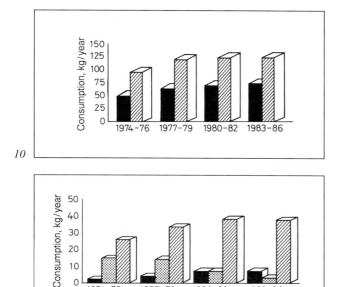

Fig. 10. Yearly per caput consumption of wheat (■) and cereals (▨).
   Fig. 11. Yearly per caput consumption of potato and tuber (■), sorghum (▥) and rice (▨).

to 46.6 g/caput/day in the mid-eighties, a steady linear increase in the consumption of animal proteins, from 15.7 g/caput/day in the mid-seventies to 37.6 g/caput/day in the mid-eighties, is a significant and expected reflection of Saudi dietary habit, and a consumption pattern associated with affluence and purchasing power (fig. 13) [51].

Daily per caput consumption of calories of animal origin showed a steady linear increase from the mid-seventies to the mid-eighties, while calories from plant sources leveled off from the early eighties to the mid-eighties. The daily consumption of total calories, as an indicator of affluence and purchasing power, both of animal and plant origin, showed a steady increase, from 1,807 kcal/caput/day in the mid-seventies to 3,012 kcal/caput/day in the mid-eighties. Calories of plant origin were the major contributors. A steady increase in the consumption of calories of animal origin is considered to be a significant turning point in the consumption

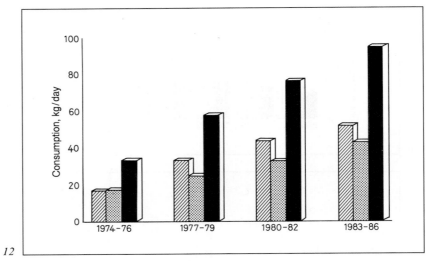

12

13

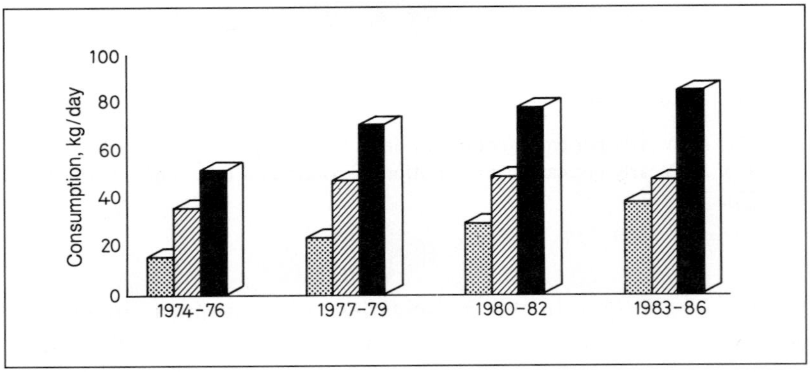

Fig. 12. Daily per caput consumption of fats of plant (▨) and animal (▦) origin. ■ = Total fats (plant and animal origin).
Fig. 13. Daily per caput consumption of protein of animal (▦) and plant (▨) origin. ■ = Total protein (animal and plant origin).

pattern associated with high purchasing power in the affluent societies (fig. 14) [51]. Recent studies are also in agreement with data presented by the Saudi Food Balance Sheets [37, 52]. A WHO report, from a situation analysis in the region, indicates a trend for increased fat consumption and decreased carbohydrate in Saudi Arabia. This trend has been going on for

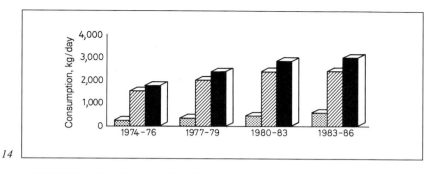

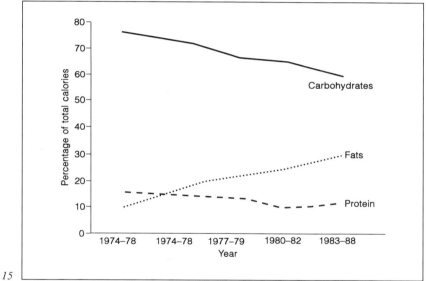

Fig. 14. Daily per caput consumption of calories of animal (▦) and plant (▨) origin. ■ = Total calories (animal and plant origin).

Fig. 15. Saudi Arabia trends in food consumption, as percent of calories available.

the last 20 years. Protein as a percentage of the total available calories has remained essentially the same in the Kingdom throughout the period of 1970 and 1986. Contribution of fats to the percentage of calories available has steadily increased, while percent calories from carbohydrates are in continuous decline (fig. 15) [37]. The average calorie and protein availability from different food categories, such as cereals, roots and tubers, pulses, fruits, vegetables and meats, showed a steady increase as well during the period of 1975 and 1984 [52].

The rapid economic development, modernization and their associated life-style have also stimulated some interest in regard to nutrient intake and dietary patterns of the vulnerable groups. Infant feeding, both breast and bottle, weaning practices and, thus, the nutritional status of children 0–72 months and older were investigated [53–55]. Al-Othaimeen et al. [53], as well as Sawaya et al. [54], have studied the feeding and weaning practices in Saudi Arabia and their relationship to the children's nutritional status. The results of these two studies provide clear evidence that rapid economic progress and modernization did not have any significant effects on breast-feeding patterns. Islamic teachings and religious beliefs advise continuing breast-feeding for up to 2 years and longer [53, 54]. A survey study, designed to investigate the nutrient intake of 849 infants and children aged 0–6 years in 4 semirural regions of Saudi Arabia, revealed a mild to moderate stunting for most age groups. Most of the babies were given powdered milk formula, the weaning foods were introduced after 6 months of age, and bottle feeding stopped after 20 months. Energy intakes were found to be below the requirements. Iron and niacin were grossly deficient despite the high values for protein [55].

Trends in Chronic Diseases

A health planning of any kind for the delivery of effective services does require baseline information, vital statistics, prevalence data, trends and future projections. In the Kingdom of Saudi Arabia, unfortunately, the lack of data and the reliability of those available have been, thus far, the major stumbling block. A recent *World Health Statistics Quarterly,* on 'Noncommunicable Diseases: A Global Problem', focused on many health problems, including those arising from dietary affluences, worldwide, with no concrete data from the Eastern Mediterranean region, except some investigations from Egypt and Kuwait [37]. Most of the data are in the form of death rates from specific diseases; the following trends in the Saudi Kingdom appear to be interesting, but need to be considered with some reservation and caution.

Obesity. The association between obesity and diabetes, hypertension, cardiovascular diseases, certain cancers, some digestive diseases and reduced life expectancy are now known and well established [4, 5, 42]. There-

Table 5. Overall prevalence of obesity among married nonpregnant females (n = 467) in Saudi Arabia [56]

Quetelet's index, kg/m^2	Cases	%	
<2	51	10.9	
20–24.9	164	35.1	
25–29.9	126	27.0	
30–34.9	88	18.8 }	27
35 and over	38	8.2 }	
Total	467	100.0	

fore, the prevalence of obesity in a general population is a rough indication of the health status as a whole. The available data clearly indicate the prevalence of adult obesity in the Kingdom, affecting women in particular. However, the data are insufficient to quantify the trend for the entire adult population [37, 38]. The risk of childhood obesity and its continuation to adulthood are now well established [6, 8, 42]. A survey, utilizing the US National Center for Health Statistic standards, carried out in the Kingdom revealed 14% childhood obesity among 0–6 years olds [37]. A study carried out by Khwaja and Al-Sibai [56] on 467 married nonpregnant Saudi female patients showed an overall prevalence of 27% obesity. Data indicated that age was a contributing factor to obesity rather than parity. A significantly higher proportion of women aged 25 years and above, as compared to those under 25 years of age, were found to be obese (table 5) [56]. The prevalence of diabetes mellitus in 1,385 Saudi males in the Al-Kharj area of Saudi Arabia was investigated using the WHO criteria for screening and interpretation of the glucose tolerance test. The prevalence was found to increase with age. The cases detected were relatively symptom-free, but 65% of the diabetic patients were overweight as compared with 26% of the nondiabetic population, and diabetes in Saudi Arabia appears to be related to obesity [57].

Similar findings were also reported by Fatani et al. [58] regarding 5,222 rural subjects of both sexes in a study of the prevalence of diabetes mellitus in the western region. The body mass index was used as an index of obesity. Men and women were considered to be obese if their body mass index was 27.0 and 25.0, respectively. Among adult subjects, 15 years and over, the rate of obesity among diabetic subjects (41.4%) was significantly

Table 6. Obesity among diabetic and nondiabetic adults in rural Saudi Arabia [58]

Subjects			Men	Women	Total
Diabetic cases	total number		69	141	210
	obese	n	27	60	87
		%	39.1	42.4	41.4
Nondiabetic cases	total number		1,646	1,315	2,901
	obese	n	351	517	868
		%	21.3	39.3	29.3

higher than that among normal subjects (29.3%). They reported that in men the obesity rate was significantly higher among diabetic subjects (39.1%) than in normal subjects (21.3%). Women did not have a significant difference in the rate of obesity between diabetic (42.4%) and normal (39.3%) subjects. The authors concluded that their results, both urban and rural, clearly show that the impact of the modernization and affluence occurring in the area over the last 2 decades has probably surfaced the problems of obesity and diabetes mellitus in a vulnerable society. The changes in life-style, i.e. diet rich in calories, sedentary life-style and urbanization, have probably contributed to the higher prevalence of obesity and diabetes (table 6) [58]. This study also showed that in normal subjects the obesity rate increased with the increase of income and was more prevalent among people of 35–54 years of age (table 7) [58]. In another study [59], the same authors have extensively investigated the patterns of complications in Saudi Arabian diabetics.

In a most recent study, Khashoggi et al. [60] looked into the factors affecting the rate of obesity among adult females in the western province of the Kingdom. According to the study, with a sample size of 950 adult females screened at primary health care centers, the prevalence of obesity is found to be correlated to age, income, marital status, parity, education, type of job, age of husband, number of servants and the availability of elevators. Other factors studied had no relation to the rate of prevalence.

Diabetes mellitus. Although diabetes mellitus in Saudi Arabia has attracted the attention of many scientists and health professionals during the last several years, only a few studies have been published [61–68].

Table 7. Obesity among diabetics and nondiabetics in Saudi Arabia according to monthly income and age [58]

Age		Low income < 3,000 SR		Average income 3,000–6,000 SR		High income > 6,000 SR	
		normal	diabetic	normal	diabetic	normal	diabetic
15–34 years							
Total number		591	10	233	8	51	10
Obese	n	29	2	66	3	15	7
	%	4.9	20.0	28.4	37.5	29.4	70.0
35–54 years							
Total number		122		74	33	15	19
Obese	n	29	20	36	28	8	14
	%	23.8	45.5	48.6	54.5	53.3	73.3
55 years and above							
Total number		161	12	31	15	25	2
Obese	n	44	1	9	8	12	1
	%	27.3	8.3	29.0	53.3	48	50.0

These studies were carried out in local communities and mostly among hospital patients. The general impression from the limited literature available is that it is an emerging problem in Saudi Arabia, particularly in urban societies. Some studies showed a relatively high prevalence of 4.5% in urban communities. It was suggested that the rapid socioeconomic changes in the country over the last 20 years must have contributed to the high prevalence rate. Many questions regarding the magnitude of the problem, its distribution, contributing factors, pathogenesis and criteria for diagnosis still need to be answered [61, 62]. Sebai [61] pointed out that populations in which diabetes is not a public health problem may show an increased incidence of diabetes as they become more affluent or their carbohydrate intake increases markedly. Apparently, this is what happened in Saudi Arabia in general, and in its urban societies in particular, as a result of the rapid socioeconomic development. Studies indicate a rather high prevalence of diabetes, 2.5% among males and 4.7% among females, in urban communities. The epidemiology of diabetes, its magnitude and the associated dietary and nutritional factors in the Kingdom have been extensively discussed by Sebai [63].

Table 8. Prevalence of diabetes mellitus in rural Saudi Arabia [58]

Age, years	Subjects studied	Subjects with diabetes	
		n	%
0–14	2,033	14	0.7
15–34	1,821	41	2.3
35–54	936	111	11.9
55 and above	432	58	13.4
Total	5,222	224	4.3

The impact of modernization and affluence on the prevalence of diabetes has been pointed out by others as well. Fatani et al. [58], studying 5,222 rural subjects of both sexes in western Saudi Arabia, looked into the parameters of blood glucose, body weight, height and socioeconomic status. The results showed an overall prevalence of 4.3% (table 8). The prevalence of diabetes differed among sexes and rose according to age and income. It was suggested from the data that the rapid socioeconomic changes in the country over the last 2 decades must have contributed to the high prevalence rates. The authors emphasized the urgent need for both health planning and education as well as the establishment of specialized centers for better management of the disease [58].

In a study covering 222 consecutive, non-insulin-dependent Saudi diabetics, the prevalence of adult-onset diabetes (85%) was similar to that of western societies [64]. The authors concluded that most diabetes in Saudi Arabia is non-insulin-dependent with onset in middle age, and patients are characteristically obese at the time of diagnosis. Polyuria, nocturia and ketosis are often absent, or mild, despite severe hyperglycemia [64]. Hagroo et al. [65], looking into the pattern of diabetes mellitus in 2,490 Saudi diabetic patients at the Riyadh Central Hospital, have noted the following characteristics among the patients examined and monitored. (1) The prevalence of non-insulin-dependent diabetes mellitus was 80.8% as compared to only 19.2% for the insulin-dependent type. (2) A special tropical type was encountered in 43.7% of the insulin-dependent diabetics. (3) Neurovascular microangiopathic complications, including diabetic foot disease, were common in all groups. The authors emphasized the importance of education and dietary management rather than insulin administration and chemotherapy for the diabetic population [65].

A recent overview of diabetes mellitus [66] concluded that the prevalence of diabetes in the Kingdom is 3–6%, and that it increases with (1) age (13% of subjects are over 55 years) and (2) socioeconomic status. Most recently, a pilot study was conducted in different regions of Saudi Arabia in order to estimate the frequency of fasting hyperglycemia in the Saudi population [67]. Most of the cases were found to be in the age range of 40 years and older. The authors proposed epidemiological studies in order to determine the prevalence of different types of diabetes, etiological factors, clinical manifestations, genetics, and the morbidity and mortality associated with diabetes in this population [67]. Recently, El-Hazmi [68] reviewed the studies reported to date for the Saudi population.

Cardiovascular Diseases and Hypertension. To date, there is no published information or reliable data indicating the prevalence of cardiovascular diseases in the Kingdom of Saudi Arabia. Data from other countries of the region suggest that these diseases are the major causes for morbidity, hospitalization and economic burden on health care services and, thus, on national development. The most reliable information concerning cardiovascular diseases is in the form of mortality data which can be extrapolated for the entire region. As reported, virtually all the countries in the region have a very high proportion of mortality from cardiovascular diseases, and for most of these countries the cardiovascular diseases have been the major causes of death. The 6 small countries in the region for which some trend information is available show an increasing incidence of deaths from cardiovascular diseases. Both Egypt and Kuwait show about 30% increases in percent mortality due to these diseases over a 10-year period. As a whole, cardiovascular diseases, both ischemic and cerebrovascular disease, show clear signs of elevation in the Kingdom of Saudi Arabia and in the entire region [37].

Cancer. One of the most recent review articles from the region states that cancer in Saudi Arabia is an ever-increasing problem as people change their life-style and longevity increases [69]. The incidence of cancer is estimated to be around 800 new cases per million population per year, as compared to 400 cases in Kuwait, 1,000 in Iraq and 4,000 in the USA. More than 70% of the cancer patients are admitted to hospitals at an advanced stage, usually beyond the curative therapy. El-Hazmi [69] expressed his concern that the care of terminally ill patients is becoming a burden in Saudi Arabia. The traditional extended family is gradually transforming into a nuclear family which makes a terminally ill cancer patient quite a big problem for both family and the government. Taking into consideration the rate of population growth, a longer life expectancy at birth, rapid industrialization, affluent life-style and the associated dietary pattern, up to 10,000 new cases of cancer per year could be expected. Therefore, as the author suggests, a balanced intervention, both preventive and curative, should be given utmost attention and priorities. The most successful approach in control of carcinogenesis lies in its prevention, but primary, avoiding the carcinogens, and secondary, with early detection and treatment [61, 69].

Several studies on cancer, mostly epidemiological, have been carried out in the Kingdom in order to determine the magnitude of the problem. In the absence of a national survey or national cancer registration, these studies are the only source of information to date on cancer in the Kingdom [69]. Mahboubi [70], reviewing the cancer profile in the Kingdom of Saudi Arabia and covering more than 11,000 cases representing the entire country, confirmed that 'a true incidence of cancer in Saudi Arabia cannot be known until a national, population-based, cancer registry is established'. The author emphasized environmental factors, such as tobacco, alcohol, snuff, carcinogens and co-carcinogens, in the etiology of cancer incidence. According to this review, the most prevalent cancer types among males are malignant (non-Hodgkin's) lymphomas and cancers of the esophagus, lung, liver and stomach; among females, breast cancer, non-Hodgkin's lymphomas, and cancers of the thyroid, esophagus and cervix prevail [70].

El-Akkad [71], in a comparative study investigating the pattern of cancer occurrences in different regions of the country, suggested that, among others, environmental, social and genetic factors may be responsible for its heterogeneous distribution in the Kingdom. In another study El-Akkad et al. [72] pointed out an upward trend in the incidence of lung, breast, colon and rectum cancer, and a downward trend in esophageal cancer; they related these trends to the rapid pace of economic progress, industrialization and affluence. Bedikian et al. [73], while investigating cancer patterns in the country, examined the psychosocial parameters and attitudes of both patients and their companions toward the disease.

Koriech and AL-Kuhaymi [74] monitored 297 patients with malignant disorders referred to the oncology unit of the Riyadh Armed Forces

Hospital, Al-Kharj, and concluded that no correlation could be established between the types of malignant disorders and any environmental, social or dietary factors, due to the small sample size. However, they could demonstrate an upward trend of bronchogenic carcinoma due to smoking and stress, as a result of rapid urbanization, sedentary life-style and industrialization. Although the etiology of esophageal cancer is not yet clearly understood, Seraj and Sabbah [75] ruled out a single factor and suggested multiple factors, involving hot spicy food, saleeg, nutritional deficiencies, environmental agents and possibly genetic factors, in the etiology, pattern and distribution of esophageal cancer.

Amer [76], monitoring 1,000 consecutive cancer patients at the King Faisal Specialist Hospital and Research Center (KFSH & RC), found that patients with gastrointestinal malignancies accounted for about 25% of all cases. He stated that such findings, even though not representing the overall incidence of cancer, may indicate that gastrointestinal malignancies, malignant lymphomas, and head and neck cancers are relatively common in the Kingdom. The importance of diet and consumption patterns in their etiology was emphasized. According to this author, dietary variables were found to be strongly correlated geographically with several types of cancer. Cancers of the breast, corpus uteri and colon have been found to be strongly associated with total protein and fat consumption, particularly meat and animal fat, while gastric cancers, and possibly head and neck cancers, have been related to malnutrition, especially the lack of vitamins. Breast cancer was reported to be more common among women of middle and upper socioeconomic status.

Changing trends in gastric cancers have been attributed to changes in dietary patterns and associated life-style practices [76]. All these studies were hospital-based; thus, results are not representative of a region or the country as a whole. Patients were, by and large, Saudis, with a small minority of non-Saudis. In the absence of a national survey or a national cancer registry these studies are the only source of information on cancer in the Kingdom of Saudi Arabia [69].

Data originating from the 'Annual Report of the Tumor Registry' of the KFSH & RC in Riyadh, a primary national referral center of excellence for specialized medical therapies and treatment of neoplastic diseases, founded in 1975, are known to be highly reliable and could be considered as a national clearinghouse reflecting all cancer cases found in the Kingdom of Saudi Arabia [77]. A total of 15,115 cancer cases were registered during the period of 1975–1987, representing 8,575 males and 6,540 females (56,7% and 43.3%, respectively; fig. 16).

16

17

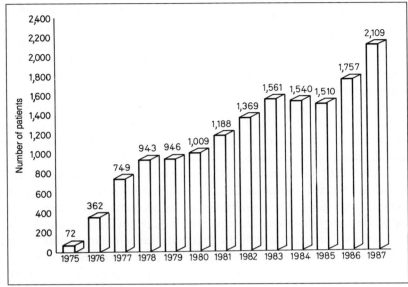

Fig. 16. Number of patients accessioned in the KFSH&RC Cancer Registry by year.

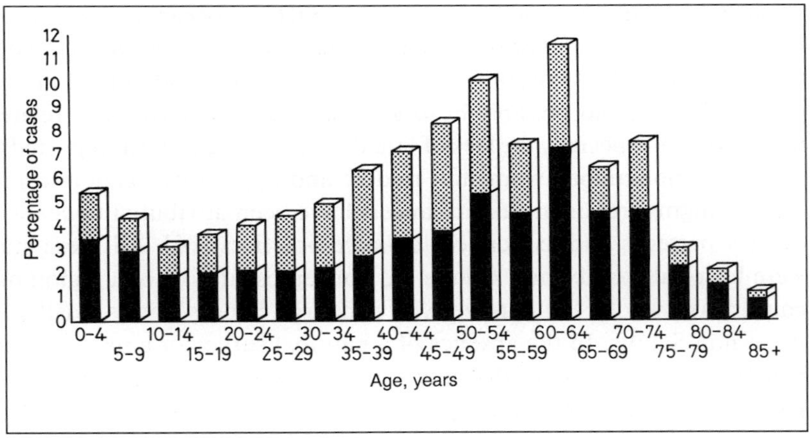

Fig. 17. Cancer distribution by age, based on 15,115 cases. ■ = Male (n = 8,575); ▒ = female (n = 8,575).

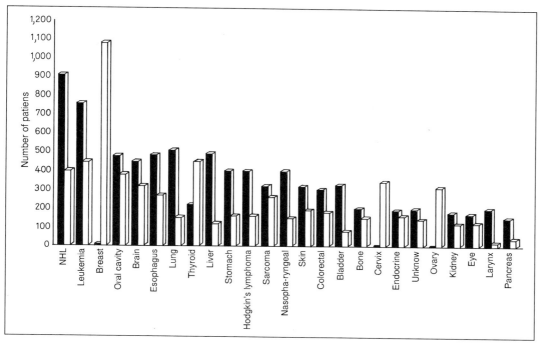

Fig. 18. Frequency of the 25 most common malignancies (1975–1987), based on 15,115 cases. ■ = Male; □ = female. NHL = Non-Hodgkin's lymphoma.

Figure 17 depicts the tumor case distribution by age. The largest number of cases occur during the 5th and 6th decades in males, and during the 4th and 5th decades in females. The frequencies of common malignancies in the Kingdom are somewhat different from those of the western world. Common tumors of the west, such as lung, colon and prostate, are much less frequent in Saudi Arabia, except for breast cancer which is just as common as in the west. Breast cancer is by far the most common tumor (16.5%) of all female malignancies. The mean age at diagnosis is a decade younger as compared to those of the west (fig. 18) [77]. All leukemias constitute the second most common neoplasm seen at the KFSH&RC. The leukemias make up the most common malignancy in children under the age of 15 years. The incidence of esophageal cancer is markedly more frequent in Saudi Arabia than in the west. The frequency of lung cancer is much lower than in western countries, indicating a much lower level of smoking and industrial pollution. It is, however, the second most common tumor in males. Colorectal cancer is markedly less common as compared to the west, for which the dietary factors may play a role. It represents 3.1% of all tumors at the KFSH&RC (fig. 18), in contrast to 15% in the west [77].

According to Sebai [61, 69, 78–80], there have been noticeable differences in the relative frequency of cancers between different regions in Saudi Arabia, reflecting the diversity of the geography, climate, urbanization, availability of health services, consumption patterns, dietary habits, educational level and life-style of people in different parts of the Kingdom. This author, in his two comprehensive reviews of the health profile in Saudi people, examined the frequencies of the most common types of cancer, their suspected etiology, the comparative health status of the selected communities (Turaba, Khulais, Tamnia, Qasim), major communicable diseases and nutritional disorders, and critically reviewed the present infrastructure of the health care services and manpower needs, both present and future, in the Kingdom of Saudi Arabia.

Oral Health and Cariogenesis. The prevalence of cariogenesis and periodontal diseases as major oral public health problems in the Gulf area has been emphasized [38]. Oral health and dental care services, as a result of rapid urbanization and socioeconomic progress, have also attracted some attention in the Kingdom by concerned health care authorities as well as by researchers. Early investigators were hampered by the lack of reliable data on the problem, and recommended in-depth and comprehensive studies [81–83]. These small-scale regional early studies, needless to say, do not reflect the national profile of Saudi Arabia. Al-Shammary and Guile [84], in the mid-eighties, presented a comprehensive outlook of dental diseases in the Kingdom, and the role of the King Saud University as a center of higher education and training in dental care services was evaluated from the viewpoint of national needs and future projections. Al-Shammary [85], in another study, stressing the role of preventive dentistry in the Kingdom, reviewed the demand for dental care in the Riyadh area. Monitoring the distribution of chief complaints by age and sex, this author pointed out that the lack of data on the prevalence of dental diseases among the Saudi population creates difficulties for planners, educators and health professionals who are involved in the dental care delivery services of the Kingdom. In a recent study, Al-Sekait and Al-Nasser [86] investigated the prevalence of dental caries in a population of 7,040 school children. The prevalence was

68%, and the DMF index (decayed, missing and filled) was 2.0. The study confirmed that caries were more prevalent in the middle- and upper-income groups, indicating the high consumption of refined sugar and sugar products. It is concluded that the application of preventive dentistry and dental education in the primary schools is the major step for the ultimate goal of a caries-free community in the Kingdom of Saudi Arabia. A most recent review article by Al-Khadra [87] also highlighted the increasing incidence of cariogenesis and dental fluorosis in certain regions due to the high fluoride content in the drinking water, and pointed out the acute shortage of dental health professionals in the country.

Guidelines and Recommendations

The following recommendations, practical guidelines and feasible projects, by and large, are the general reflection of the consensus reached by the delegates representing the countries of the Eastern Mediterranean Region (EMRO/WHO) on the issues and problems of the affluent diet and consumption patterns during a regional meeting which was held in Nicosia, Cyprus, in May 1989 [37].

The Advocacy: Administrative and Political Support

Food abundance, excessive caloric intake and overnutrition have traditionally been considered as the blessings of Allah, and have never been looked upon as alarming factors until recently when our planet gradually plunged itself into the so-called diseases of civilization because of our sedentary living pattern, push-button life-style and the affluent diet. It is about time, and in fact a little too late, that the national health authorities through a concerted effort and the cooperation of the UN organizations, such as the WHO and others, organize themselves for the development of major guidelines and public health policies concerning the consequences of excessive caloric intake and overconsumption. Needless to say, these chronic killer diseases and clinical entities have always been in the hands of curative medicine and will remain so unless major steps forward are taken in order to create public awareness, through mass education, for their feasible preventability.

As far as the public opinion and responses are concerned, the lack of awareness and shortage of information have been the major stumbling blocks. Therefore, it is the major responsibility of the health profession-

als, academies, scientists and above all the media to advocate and dramatize these stark realities, with facts, figures and other documentation, and
bring them to the attention of government authorities, planners and deci-
sion makers so that they will be sensitized enough to draw political and
administrative support for legislative actions. It is through these channels
and proper legislative actions that the local and national governments
could lay down the foundation for the development of guidelines and public policies in order to alleviate the disastrous consequences of these
chronic and degenerative diseases due to our sedentary life-style, overconsumption and the affluent diet.

The Administrative Unit: The Infrastructure

An administrative unit, either at the ministerial cabinet level or within
a ministry of health, should be established as a leader of the national
infrastructure for the coordination of the above criteria and activities.
Such a centrally located administrative unit and its supportive functional
linkages should be the essential part of any national network, and will be in
charge of all kinds of food and nutrition planning activities, both preventive and curative, for the regions in question.

As an example, the infrastructure of the Department of Nutrition
within the ministry of Health of the Kingdom of Saudi Arabia and its
major components are presented in figure 19 [88, 89]. Through an effective
national network extending to each Health Directorate, the Department of
Nutrition is in operation in order to manage and monitor the community
activities in 18 Health Directorates through the 'Community Nutrition
Unit', which controls the Primary Health Care Centers, and the 'Nutrition
and Dietary Services Unit' under each hospital administration throughout
the Kingdom. In addition to its major divisions, the Scientific and Technical Advisory Committee, a standing active unit within the department,
monitors project identifications, developments and implementations in
research, training and extension activities throughout the Kingdom of
Saudi Arabia.

Intersectoral Food and Nutrition Planning Council

It is now a widely recognized and well-established fact that the science
of nutrition is a multidisciplinary subject; its projects and programs
require multiskilled coordination and intersectoral approach for their
effective implementation. Being multisectoral in nature and character,
nutritional issues and problems need coordination of the comprehensive

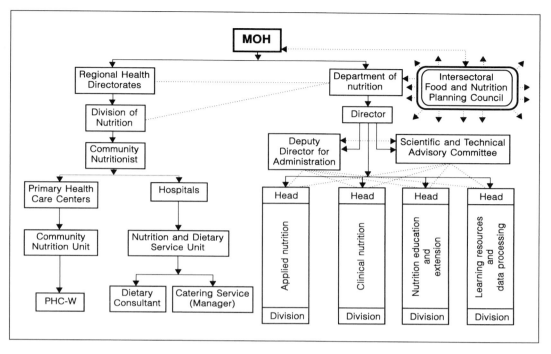

Fig. 19. Infrastructure of the Department of Nutrition, Ministry of Health (MOH), Kingdom of Saudi Arabia [88].

strategies and policies within the framework of national development. Thus, the health sector, or any other sector alone, would not be able to have any effective impact on the nutritional status of a given population. Therefore, the necessity for the formation of a coordinated, multiskilled and multisectoral committee or council appears to be inevitable. Such unit, or body, under titles such as 'national food and nutrition planning council or committee' is now a common household word in many countries. The health sector, i.e. a ministry of health, because of its unique position, has an important role within this multisectoral framework. Thus, it should take a leadership role for the formation of an 'intersectoral food and nutrition planning council' for national programs, policies and development strategies. Figure 19 reflects the relative position of such a council under the leadership of the Ministry of Health, Kingdom of Saudi Arabia.

National Food and Nutrition Policies

Political support, the administrative infrastructure and the establishment of a national center or department of nutrition and its essential components are all major achievements which are required for the development of national food and nutrition policies and their effective implementation in any given nation [89]. The intersectoral food and nutrition planning council, under the leadership of the national administrative unit, a department of nutrition, should respond to all issues and problems related to food and nutrition, both under- and overnutrition, for the development of national dietary guidelines and policies [90].

Development of National Dietary Guidelines

The US and several other western countries have already developed national dietary guidelines for their citizens and have been guiding them for proper dietary patterns and life-style. Some nations went even further to regionalize these dietary guidelines and recommendations. Once the national infrastructure is being firmly established, then dietary guidelines, similar to those of western nations, based on local and regional traditions, food preferences, consumption habits and life-style, should be developed as part of the national food and nutrition programs and policies, and be put into practice and closely monitored [90]. In the Kingdom of Saudi Arabia, these dietary guidelines could be implemented by both the hospitals and the primary health care centers in the regionalized communities. This is feasible and can easily be done by proper training, national coordination and international cooperation.

Mass Media and Public Awareness

The role of media (press, radio, TV) for the creation of mass public awareness toward the consequences of our life-style and eating habits is extremely vital and requires individual cooperation. Nutritional education, as a component of general health education and personal hygiene, through primary, secondary and university levels, is indeed the most effective channel for transmitting basic health information to the young generation which will have a lasting effect during their adulthood. School systems, at any level, could be the most ideal vehicles in order to accomplish these objectives.

In the Kingdom of Saudi Arabia, with close cooperation and coordination with the Ministry of Health, the Ministry of Education should take the leadership role of coordinating an 'inter-school board' in order to review, evaluate and implement an 'action-oriented school health and nutrition education curriculum' at all levels, including vocational and Koranic schools. Similarly, a package of 'family health education' components should be established in every primary health care center, should include a series of video cassettes on malnutrition modules, both undernutrition and overnutrition, and should constitute a part of the compulsory 'family education programs' during their visit to the Primary Health Care Centers for the required immunizations. Such video cassettes with health education models should include subjects such as oral rehydration therapy, growth monitoring, breast-feeding, immunizations, communicable diseases and family planning, and be checked out by the families and followed up by the primary health care workers in their respective communities.

Nutritional Support Unit in Primary Health Care Centers, Clinics and Hospitals

As a support to mass media and public awareness programs and campaigns, it is recommended that medical practices and diagnostic services in the primary health care centers, clinics and hospitals should exercise preventive and promotional activities, in parallel with curative ones. These preventive and promotional activities should include a basic and comprehensive assessment of the nutritional status, dietary counseling and health education including behavior modification as related to eating habits and life-style. These services should be community-oriented and designed to create public awareness through individual counseling. Although certain hospitals and clinics such as the KFSH&RC do have such facilities, they should be more comprehensive and nationwide, and should include primary health care centers as well. In short, principles and guidelines of preventive medicine and health promotional activities should be introduced and made part of the curative health care services. It is also recommended that the dietary services in the Kingdom's hospitals be evaluated and upgraded from the viewpoints of manpower, ethics, services and training.

Role of the Food Industry

Throughout the history of science and technology, food science, from its early primitive stage to the most sophisticated levels of our time, has played a unique and significant role in the nourishment of mankind. National coordination and partnerships, which have been established between industry, private sectors, academies and governments, and the regulatory agencies, have been and will always be the vital determining

factor in future advances and progress. The contributions of this strategic
partnership have been in many aspects of food sciences and technology,
such as food hygiene and safety, quality control, processing, preservation,
enrichment, fortification, labeling and genetic engineering, just to name a
few. All these frontiers, in one way or another, have contributed to better
nourishment of human populations everywhere. Simopoulos [91] emphasized the fact that food sciences and technology will be guided and directed
by our expanding knowledge of nutritional sciences which influence
directly or indirectly health, diseases and the genetic variations of the
human population. This author pointed out the necessity for the creation
of a national 'nutrition and food sciences agency' which will have to 'co-
habitate' and work in harmony for future progress in food sciences, nutrition research, education and extension. New national programs, policies
and relevant guidelines, within the framework of this partnership, must be
developed in order to deal effectively with the consequences of malnutrition, and such a national or federal agency should assume major responsi-
bilities in their strategic implementations [91].

Target-Oriented Education, Training, Extension and Research Activities

A cadre of properly trained health workers is an integral part of any
health care delivery services. Training provision of knowledge where it is
needed the most should be the motto of a health care system which gears
itself for prevention, early detection, treatment, rehabilitation and health
promotion. Therefore, the training of the health professionals, at all levels,
should be given the utmost priority. The required 'nutrition manpower'
including community and clinical nutritionists as well as dietitians who are
qualified to deal with all aspects of nutritional sciences, is a *must*. Plans are
now underway to include 'nutrition education' curricula as part of the
required school health education programs in elementary, secondary and
vocational schools, and at higher education levels throughout the Kingdom. The need for nutrition education in the general population could be
effectively addressed through the school systems. Eating habits and consumption patterns are generally set during these formative years. Proper
diet and eating habits during childhood and adolescence could have the
effect of helping to prevent nutrition-related problems later in life. The
Ministry of education of the Kingdom of Saudi Arabia is responsible for
nutrition education and introduction of nutrition curricula throughout the
system of education, at all levels.

It is also critical that physicians, nurses, dietitians and other health professionals be aware of the nutritional status of a community or of a patient in order to launch sound intervention and therapeutic programs. This can only be accomplished by the introduction of formal training programs into the curricula of health sciences in both preventive and curative medicine [92]. Therefore, medical schools, throughout the Kingdom of Saudi Arabia, should reconsider the priorities of what will be taught within the available time, provide financial support and make every possible effort to achieve the goals of an adequate level of nutrition education for all health professionals [92]. It has already been recommended that a task force should be established in order to carry out a feasibility study for the establishment of a school of public health under one of the university systems in order to respond and satify the national health needs and objectives. Such academic institutions will eventually serve the entire Middle-East for the required manpower in preventive and promotional health care services [61, 88].

To date, the lack of reliable data and documentation on a variety of health problems, such as regional and national nutritional status, deficiencies, diet and life-style-related chronic killer diseases, hamper the development and implementation of effective target-oriented intervention programs for the population groups in question. A nationwide survey, 'Health and Nutritional Status of the Saudi People', has already been undertaken and is well in progress. This national project, when it is completed, will provide solid baseline data for numerous target-oriented action programs and projects in research, training and extension activities.

The Ultimate: You, the Individual

We are *not* all born equal, at least, not as far as our health is concerned. Our attitudes toward health and life-style, which shape and mold our personality and physical well-being, are the major determining factors for the welfare and quality of our life. One must keep in mind that the seeds of many of our adult health problems are showed during childhood and the formative years. Eating and consumption patterns, physical activities and exercise habits and exposure to carcinogens could have profound and long-lasting effects on our health. We can, however, do a great deal about our health and well-being, and promote welfare. Most of our serious health problems are directly or indirectly related to our personal habits, life-style and behaviors, such as drug abuse, smoking, sedentary pattern of work, stress, lack of exercise, poor eating habits and overconsumption, just to name a few.

The health care industry, worldwide, is designed and developed to serve and care for the morbids, because we only think about health when we are sick and not feeling well. The best time, however, to think about our health is *before* we get sick. Better health and well-being are not just a matter of luck or fate. We can and must do something about it. As once stated by Joseph Califano, the former Secretary of Health and Human Services of the US Government, during the Carter administration:

'... You, the individual, can do more for your own health and well-being than any doctor, any hospital, any drug, and any exotic medical device ...'.

Yes, indeed, we can and *must* do, through changes in life-style and behavior modification, necessary changes to alleviate the profound consequences of overnutrition. As Simopoulos [93] underline, proper nutrition and fitness should be part of the physician's armamentarium in the control of chronic diseases as they afflict our society today. An increase in physical activity along with a decrease in total energy intake and a decrease in dietary fat are needed to control obesity in sedentary affluent societies [93].

However, governments, through the help and cooperation of international health organizations, have the responsibility to provide both a structure of incentives and a source of information in order to motivate and enhance the general well-being of their population. Just like the programs, policies and interventions throughout the sixties and seventies were formulated and implemented in order to combat undernutrition and alleviate its miseries and consequences, now it is about time that every government, both developing and developed, take a new direction and a step forward in the formulation of public health policies, nutritional goals and programs, and spell out new dietary guidelines for the prevention of these chronic and degenerative killer diseases due to our hazardous life-style, dietary habits and overconsumption [2, 90].

Acknowledgments

Thanks and appreciation are due to the senior members of the Department for their interest and continuous support, to Dr. N.H. Ozerol for the editorial touch, and to Mr. Khan Mosharref Hussain and Mr. A. Samad for their assistance in the preparation of the computerized illustrations and the outstanding secretarial work.

References

1 Eckholm E, Record F: The two faces of malnutrition. Worldwatch Paper No 9. Washington, Worldwatch Institute, 1976, pp 23–48.

2 Eckholm E, Record F: The affluent diet: A worldwide health hazard. Futurist 1977; 11:19–25.

3 Heart Disease: Public Health Enemy No 1. Hearings before the Subcommittee on Nutrition of the Committee on Agriculture, Nutrition and Forestry. United States Senate, 69th Congress, 1st session, May 1977.

4 McGinnis JM, Mario N: The Surgeon General's Report on Nutrition and Health: Policy implications and implementation strategies. Am J Clin Nutr 1989;49:23–28.

5 The role of nutrition in disease prevention and health promotion and maintenance. Nutr News 1985;48:13–16.

6 The Surgeon General's Report on Nutrition and Health. USDHHS (PHS) Publ No 88–50210. Washington, US Government Printing Office 1988.

7 Beaton GH: Nutritional problems of affluence. Nutrition in Preventive Medicine, annex 2, 1976, pp 482–499.

8 Bray GA (ed): Obesity in America. USDHEW/PHS. NIH Publ No 79–359. Bethesda, National Institutes of Health, 1979, pp 34–36.

9 Levy BT, Williamson PS: Patient perceptions and weight loss of obese adults. J Fam Pract 1988;27:285–290.

10 Diet and Coronary Heart Disease. Washington, Food and Nutrition Board of the National Academy of Science, and Council on Food and Nutrition of the American Medical Association, 1972.

11 Report on the Epidemiology, Control and Management of Coronary Heart Disease in Nepal. New Delhi, WHO, 1974.

12 Stamler R, Stamler J, Riedlinger WF, et al: Weight and blood pressure: FIndings in hypertension screening of one million Americans. JAMA 1978;240:1607–1610.

13 Frohlich E: The national high blood pressure programmes. J Am Coll Cardiol 1988; 12:812–813.

14 Isaacson LC: Sodium intake and hypertension. Lancet 1963;i:946–949.

15 Tobian L Jr: Dietary salt (sodium) and hypertension. Am J Clin Nutr 1979; 32:2659–2662.

16 Zemel MB, Sowers JR: Salt sensitivity and systemic hypertension in the elderly. Am J Cardiol 1988;61:7–12.

17 Henry RR, Breachtel G, Griver K: Secretion and hepatic extraction of insulin after weight loss in obese non-insulin-dependent diabetes mellitus. J Clin Endocrinol Metab 1988;66:979–986.

18 Anderson JW, Gustafson NJ, Bryant CA, et al: Dietary fiber and diabetes: A comprehensive review and practical applications. J Am Diet Assoc 1987;87:1189–1197.

19 Nuttal FQ: Dietary recommendations for individuals with diabetes mellitus. Am J Clin Nutr 1980;33:1311–1312.

20 Ekoe JM: Diabetes mellitus: Aspects of the Worldwide Epidemiology of Diabetes mellitus and Its Long-Term Complications. New York, Elsevier, 1988.

21 Shimkin MB: Diet and Cancer. USDHHS/PHS. NIH Publ No 84–568, Bethesda, National Institutes of Health, 1983, pp 35–88.

22 Boice JD: Cancer following medical irradiation (abstract). National Cancer Institute. Environmental Epidemiology Branch. Radiation Studies Section. Natl Conf on Cancer Prevention and Detection, Chicago. New York, American Cancer Society, 1980.

23 Shils ME: Nutritional and dietary factors in neoplastic development; in Nutrition and Cancer. New York, American Cancer Society, 1972, pp 1–9.

24 Wydner EL: Dietary habits and cancer epidemiology. Proc Am Cancer Soc Natl Cancer Inst. Natl Conf on Nutrition in Cancer. Cancer 1979;43:1955–1961.

25 Hegsted DM: Optimal nutrition. Cancer 1979;43:1996–2003.

26 Gori GB: Diet and cancer. J Am Diet Assoc 1977;71:375–379.

27 Weinhouse S. The role of diet and nutrition and cancer. Cancer 1986;58:1791–1794.

28 Sidney S, Farquhar JW: Cholesterol, cancer and public health policy. Am J Med 1983;75:494–508.

29 Palmer S, Bakshi K: Diet, nutrition and cancer: Interim dietary guidelines. J Natl Cancer Inst 1983;70:1151–1170.

30 Hutter RV: Cancer prevention and detection: Status report and future prospects. Cancer 1988;61:2372–2378.

31 Purtilo DT, Cohen SM: Diet, nutrition and cancer. An update on a controversial relationship. Postgrad Med 1985;78:193–203.

32 Mumford S: Nutrition and high fiber diet. Nurs Mirror 1985;160:36–38.

33 Hill MJ: Colon cancer: A disease of fiber depletion of or dietary excess. Digestion 1974;2:289–292.

34 Hill MJ, Hawksworth G, Tattersall G: Bacteria, nitrosamines and cancer of the stomach. Br J Cancer 1973;28:562–575.

35 Shubik P: Food additives. Cancer 1979;43:1982–1986.

36 Food and Nutrition Broad, Division of Biological Sciences, Assembly of Life Sciences, National Research Council: Toward healthful diets. Washington, National Academy of Sciences, 1980.

37 Clinical disorders arising from dietary affluence in countries of the eastern Mediterranean region: Situation analysis and guidelines for control. Tech Publ No 14. WHO/EMRO, Alexandria, 1989.

38 Musaiger AO: The state of food and nutrition in the Arabian Gulf countries; in Bourne GH: Nutrition in the Gulf Countries. Malnutrition and Minerals. World Rev Nutr Diet. Basel, Karger, 1987, vol 54, pp 105–173.

39 Subcommittee on nutrition, Administrative Committe on Coordination: First Report on the World Nutrition Situation. New York, United Nations, 1987, pp 27–29.

40 Farrag OI: The state of child nutrition in the Gulf Arab states. J Trop Pediatr 1983;29:325–329.

41 Amine EK, Al-Awaidi F, Rabie M: Infant feeding pattern and weaning practices in Kuwait. Abstr Symp on Nutrition. Riyadh, King Faisal Specialist Hospital and Research Center, 1989.

42 Health Implications of Obesity. Consensus Development Conference Statement No. 5. Bethesda, National Instiues of Health, 1985, pp 1–14.

43   Al-Awaidi F, Amine EK: A study of factors affecting the prevalence of obesity among adult females in Kuwait. Abstr Symp on Nutrition. Riyadh, King Faisal Specialist Hospital and Research Center, 1989.

44   Department of Economic Studies and Statistics: Food Balance Sheets. Jeddah, Ministry of Agriculture and Water, Kingdom of Saudi Arabia, 1987.

45   El-Khatib AB: Seven Green Spikes ed 2. Jeddah, Ministry of Agriculture and Water, Kingdom of Saudi Arabia. 1980 pp 11–50.

46   Gardner GR: Saudi Arabia's drive for agricultural self-sufficiency: A political goal with high economic costs. Middle East and Africa. Outlook and Situation Report. Economic Research Service RS 85–3. USDA-USA, 1985.

47   Gardner GR: Saudi food imports: A case of the permanent income hypothesis at work. Middle East and North Africa. Outlook and Situation Report. Economic Research Service RS 86–1. USDA-USA, 1986.

48   Gardner GR: Saudi Arabia to promote barley production, reduce wheat surplus. World agricultural highlists. Economic Research Service RS 29–86. USDA-USA, 1986.

49   Gardner GR: Saudi Arabia's agricultural sector: Impressive performance, high costs, and tough policy options. Paper presented at the Annual Meeting of the Middle East Studies Association, Boston, 1986.

50   Central Department of Statistics: Nutrition in the Kingdom of Saudi Arabia. National Nutrition Statistics. Jeddah, Ministry of Finance and National Economy, Kingdom of Saudi Arabia, 1982, pp 7–47.

51   Department of Economic Studies and Statistics: Saudi Arabian Food Balance Sheets from 1974–1976 to 1983–1986. Ministry of Agricultural and Water, Kingdom of Saudi Arabia, 1988, vol 2, pp 101–117.

52   Al-Mokhalalati JK: Development of nutritional adequacy and health status in Saudi Arabia. Saudi Med J 1989;11:18–24.

53   Al-Othaimeen AI, Villanueva BP, Devol EB: The present trend in infant feeding practices in Saudi Arabia. Food Nutr Bull 1987;9:62–68.

54   Sawaya WN, Tannous RI, Al-Othaimeen AI, et al: Breast feeding practices in Saudi Arabia. Food Nutr Bull 1987;9:69–72.

55   Al-Othaimeen AI, Sawaya WN, Tannous RI, et al: A nutrition survey of infants and preschool children in Saudi Arabia. Saudi Med J 1988;9:40–48.

56   Khwaja SS, Al-Sibai H: The relationship of age and parity to obesity in Saudi female patients. Saudi Med J 1987;8:35–39.

57   Bacchus RA, Bell JL, Madkour M, et al: The prevalence of diabetes mellitus in male Saudi Arabs. Diabetologia 1982;23:330–332.

58   Fatani HH, Mira SA, El-Zubeir AG: Prevalence of diabetes mellitus in rural Saudi Arabia. Diabetes Care 1987;10:180–187.

59   Fatani HH, Mira SA, El-Zubei AG: The pattern of complications in Saudi Arabian diabetics. Ann Saudi Med 1989;9:44–47.

60   Khashoggi RH, Madani KA, Ghaznawy HI, et al: A study of factors affecting the prevalence of obesity among adult females in Saudi Arabia. Abstr First Saudi Symp on Food. Riyadh, King Saudi University, 1990.

61   Sebai ZA: Health in Saudi Arabia. Riyadh, Directorate of Scientific Research, King Abdul Aziz City for Science and Technology, 1987, vol 2, pp 127–159.

62   Sebai ZA: Diabetes mellitus in Saudi Arabia; thesis. Middle East 1987;10:582-
      586.
63   Sebai ZA: Diabetes mellitus in Saudi Arabia. Health Dev Int Symp on Diabetes
      mellitus in Saudi Arabia. Ann Saudi Med 1987; 7: 7–8.
64   Kingston M, Skoog WC: Diabetes in Saudi Arabia. Saudi Med J 1986;7:130–142.
65   Hagroo A, Sadiq M, Al-Khawaji MZ, et al: Pattern of Diabetes mellitus in Saudi
      Arabia. Symp on Diabetes mellitus in Saudi Arabia. Riyadh, Medical City, King
      Fahad National Guard Hospital, 1986.
66   Ahmed M: An overview of Diabetes mellitus in the Kingdom of Saudi Arabia. Abstr
      Symp on Nutrition. Riyadh, King Faisal Specialist Hospital and Research Center,
      1989.
67   El-Hazmi MAF, Warsy AS: A comparative study of hyperglycemia in different
      regions of Saudi Arabia. Ann Saudi Med 1989;9:435–438.
68   El-Hazmi MAF: Diabetes mellitus – Present state of art. Saudi Med J 1990;11:
      10–17.
69   Sebai ZA: Cancer in Saudi Arabia. Ann Saudi Med 1989;9:55–63.
70   Mahboubi E: Epidemiology of cancer in Saudi Arabia. Ann Saudi Med 1987;7:
      265–276.
71   El-Akkad SM: Cancer in Saudi Arabia: A comparative study. Saudi Med J 1983;4:
      156–164.
72   El-Akkad SM, Amer MH, Sabbah RS, et al: Pattern of cancer in Saudi Arabs referred
      to King Faisal Specialist Hospital. Cancer 1986;58:1172–1178.
73   Bedikian AY, Saleh V, Ibrahim S: Saudi patient and companion attitudes toward
      cancer. King Faisal Specialist Hosp Med J 1985;5:17–25.
74   Koriech OM, Al-Kuhaymi R: Cancer in Saudi Arabia: Riyadh, Al-Kharj hospital
      programme experience. Saudi Med J 1984;5:217–223.
75   Seraj AA, Sabbah D: Carcinoma of the esophagus in Saudi Arabia. 1983;4:313–
      316.
76   Amer MH: Pattern of cancer in Saudi Arabia: A personal expeience based on the
      management of 1000 patients. Part I. King Faisal Specialist Hosp Med J 1982;2:
      203–215.
77   Annual Report of the Tumor Registry. Riyadh, King Faisal Specialist Hospital and
      Research Center, 1988.
78   Sebai ZA: Health in Saudi Arabia. Tihama, 1985, vol 1, pp 181–238.
79   Sebai ZA: Nutritional disorders in Saudi Arabia: A review. Fam Pract 1987;5:56–
      61.
80   Sebai ZA: Community Health in Saudi Arabia. A Profile of Two Villages in Qassim
      Region. Saudi Med J Monogr 1982;1:1–110.
81   El-Angabawi MF, Younes SA: Periodontal disease prevalence, and dental needs
      among school children in Saudi Arabia. Dent Oral Epidemiol 1982;10:98–99.
82   Younes SA, El-Angbawi MF: Dental caries prevalence in intermediate Saudi school
      children in Riyadh. Community Dent Oral Epidemiol 1982;10:74–76.
83   Salem GM, Holm SA: Dental caries in preschool children in Gizan, Saudi Arabia.
      Community Dent Oral Epidemiol 1985;13:176–180.
84   Al-Shammary AR, Guile EE: The dental health system of Saudi Arabia. Odontosto-
      matology 1986;9:235–238.

85   Al-Shammary AR: Demand for dental care in Saudi Arabia. Ann Saudi Med 1987;7: 327–329.

86   Al-Sekait MA, Al-Nasser AN: Dental caries prevalence in primary Saudi school children in Riyadh district. Saudi Med J 1988;9:606–609.

87   Al-Khadra BH: Dental health and health care in Saudi Arabia. Ann Saudi Med 1989; 9:592–596.

88   Al-shoshan AA: Towards a National Nutrition Policy: Proposed Plan of Actions. Riyadh, Department of Nutrition, Ministry of Health, Kingdom of Saudi Arabia, 1989.

89   Al-Shoshan AA: Towards a National Nutrition Policy. Abstr First Saudi Symp on Food. Riyadh, King Saud University. 1990.

90   Scrimshaw NS: Nutritional Goals and Dietary Guidelines for Health. Abstr First Saudi Symp on Food. Riyadh, King Saud University, 1990.

91   Simopoulos AP: The future direction of nutrition research: A nutrition and food sciences agency is the key to progress. J Nutr 1989;119:137–139.

92   Ozerol NH: Nutritional assessment: Its significance in medical education. J Med Educ 1982;57:1491–1492.

93   Simopoulos AP: Nutrition and fitness. JAMA 1989;261:2862–2863.

Ahmed A. Al-shoshan, MSc, PhD, Department of Nutrition,
King Saud University, Ministry of Health, Riyadh (Saudi Arabia)

Subject Index

Alcohol, intake effects
  diabetes 24
  obesity 17
Amino acids, dietary effect on beta cell function 24
γ-Aminobutyric acid
  hypertension role 55
  vitamin B_6 deficiency effect on level 42, 45, 50

Calcium
  dietary effects on hypertension 57–63
  effect on influx
    vitamin B_6 deficiency 55–60
    vitamin D 62
  levels in hypertensives 62, 63
  nifedipine effects on arterial tone 56
  regulation disturbance as hypotension cause 55
Cancer
  affluent diet association 118
  dietary fat effects 118
  food additive effects 118, 119
  Saudi Arabia
    age distribution 150, 151
    incidence 147, 148, 151, 152
    types correlated with affluence 148, 149
Carbohydrates, dietary
  effect
    diabetes
      mortality 18
      refined sugar 19
      soluble fiber 20
      starch 19, 20

glucose levels 18
insulin sensitivity 18
refined sugar consumption in industrialized nations 115
Cholecalciferol, *see* Vitamin D
Clonidine
  antihypertensive drug 50
  mechanism of action 50–52
  vitamin B_6 deficiency effects
    antihypertensive effects 50, 51
    receptor binding 50, 51
Coronary heart disease
  affluent diet association 116, 117
  incidence 116
  mortality 116, 117

Diabetes, non-insulin dependent
  affluent diet association 117, 118
  diagnosis 2
  diet effects
    alcohol 24
    carbohydrates 18
    fat 20–23
    meat consumption 21
    micronutrients 24, 25
    protein 23, 24
  etiology role
    age 4
    alcohol intake 24, 25
    body fat distribution 13–15
    diet 17–25
    glucose tolerance impairment 12
    heredity 3, 4
    hyperinsulinemia 2, 3, 15, 16

Diabetes, etiology role (continued)
    hypertension 11
    insulin resistance 2, 3, 15, 16
    obesity 1–17, 25, 143–145
    physical activity 6, 7, 25
    serum cholesterol 11
    smoking 11, 17, 25
  exercise effect on insulin resistance 13
  incidence 7–10, 117, 124, 125, 145–147
  mortality reduced during food shortages 5
  prevalence association with mean body
    weight in cross-cultural studies 5–10, 117
  prevention 117, 118
  syndrome X relationship 2, 4, 23
Diet
  Middle East
    affluent diet composition 123, 124
    calorie consumption trends 121, 122
    demographics 119, 120
    diet components 121, 122
    food
      adulteration 123
      production 119–121
    prevalence
      alcohol consumption 125
      cancer 126
      cardiovascular mortality 125
      diabetes 124, 125
      hypertension 125, 126
      obesity 124
      oral disease 126
      smoking 125
  most commonly chosen foods 130, 131
  overnutrition, *see also* Obesity
    description of diet 114, 115
    form of malnutrition 113, 114
    global trends 114–119
  quality measurement 132
  Saudi Arabia
    agricultural problems 129
    Department of Nutrition infrastructure
      154, 155
    diet
      development of national guidelines
        156
      education roles
        food industry 157, 158
        government 158, 159
        hospitals 157
        individual citizens 159, 160
        mass media 156, 157

    quality
      age effects 135
      education effects 133
      measurement 132
      residence effects 133–135
      food imports 128, 129
    food
      most commonly chosen foods 130,
        131, 134–136
      production trends 127, 128
      self-sufficiency program 126–128
    infant feeding 142
    intersectoral food and nutrition planning
      council 154, 155
    meal frequency 131, 132, 136
    Multipurpose Household Survey 129,
      130
    per capita consumption trends
      animal products 136–141
      carbohydrates 141
      cereals 137–139
      fats and oils 137–141
      fruits and vegetables 137, 138
      protein 141
      rice 138, 139
    percentage of residents on special diet
      135, 136
    prevalence
      cancer 147–152
      diabetes 144–147
      hypertension 147
      obesity 142–144
      oral disease 152, 153
    programs to prevent overnutrition 153,
      154

Eicosapentaenoic acid, *see* Fatty acids

Fat, dietary
  diabetes mellitus risk factor 20, 21
  effect
    cancer incidence 118
    carbohydrate metabolism 20, 21
    diabetes incidence 21–23
  percent of affluent diet 115
Fatty acids
  eicosapentaenoic acid
    cholesterol ester incorporation 102, 103
    diet effects
      blood pressure 85, 105
      hyperlipemics
        apolipoprotein levels 98, 104

blood pressure 98, 99
cholesterol level 97
free fatty acids 97
lipoprotein distribution 95
serum triglycerides 96
hypertensives
blood pressure 91–93, 99–101
eicosapentaenoic acid content in
lipids 99, 100
heart rate 92, 93
lipoprotein distribution 93, 94,
100–102
thromboxane B_2 levels 92, 94, 102,
105, 106
lipoprotein distribution 84, 85, 89–91
mackerel vs herring diet 89–91, 103
dietary linolenic acid effect on levels
75–83
metabolism 84, 85
sources 84, 85, 89
free fatty acid effects
glucose metabolism 15
hyperinsulinemia induction 15, 16
lipoprotein metabolism 16
linolenic acid
conversion to eicosapentaenoic acid diet
effects 75, 76, 83
dietary effects
blood pressure 80, 81, 83, 84
serum lipid distribution
hyperlipemics 78–82
hypertensives 78–82
metabolic pathway 76
slow in humans 77
α-linolenic acid
conversion to arachidonic acid
diet effects 75, 76, 83
metabolic pathway 76
slow in humans 77
dietary effects
blood pressure 80, 81, 83, 84
hyperlipemics 78–82
hypertensives 78–82
ω3 fatty acids
complement to vegetable oils in diet
103
dietary effects
blood pressure 85, 105
diabetes incidence 22, 23, 26
eicosanoid production 22
glucose intolerance 22
liver 104

membrane fluidity 23, 26
mechanism of hypertension protection
105, 106
metabolic fate 102, 103
methods of increasing levels in diets 106
structural features related to benefits
107
polyunsaturated fatty acids, measurement
of beneficial effects 75
Fiber, diet effects on glucose intolerance 20, 26

Hypertension
animal models 44–46, 49
anticonvulsant drug effects in vitamin B_6
deficiency 47
clonidine effects 50–52
diabetes risk factor 11
dietary effects 41
dietary salt relationship 117
eicosapentaenoic acid
content in lipids 99, 100
dietary effects
blood pressure 91–93, 99–101
heart rate 92, 93
lipoprotein distribution 93, 94,
100–102
thromboxane B_2 levels 92, 94, 102,
105, 106
etiology 41
hypothyroidism correlation 42, 43, 47
incidence 40, 125, 126, 147
role
γ-aminobutyric acid 55
calcium 55–60
norepinephrine 48–52
serotonin 52
vitamin D 64
treatment 40, 41
vitamin B_6 effects 43–50

Middle East, see Diet

Norepinephrine
hypertension role 48–52
vitamin B_6 effects
heart, turnover rate 49
myocardial content 49
plasma levels 48

Obesity
affluent diet association 115, 116
body fat distribution

Obesity (continued)
    diabetes risk factor 13–15
    intra-abdominal fat as diabetes predictor
        14, 15
    measurement 13
  diabetes mellitus etiology role 1–17, 25,
    143, 144
  effects
    alcohol 17
    smoking 17
  energy imbalance indicator 4
  glucose
    intolerance risk factor 4, 6, 10, 11
    level variance with body weight 12, 13
  history of acceptance 116
  hyperinsulinemia association 6
  incidence 116, 124, 142–144
  insulin sensitivity
    determinants
      alcohol intake 17
      exercise 17
      genetics 16
      hormones 16, 17
    role 15
  physical activity relationship 7, 11
ω fatty acids, *see* Fatty acids

Parathyroid hormone
  calcium
    homeostasis role 60, 61
    regulation of hormone levels 63, 64
  hypertension role 61
Protein, dietary effect on glucose intolerance
  23, 24
Pyridoxine, *see* Vitamin B_6

Serotonin
  receptor
    effects on hypertension
      agonist 53–55
      antagonist 54
    functions 52, 53
  vitamin B_6 effects on level 45, 50, 52
Syndrome X, diabetes relationship 2, 4, 23

Thromboxane B_2
  blood pressure effects 106
  dietary fish oil effect on levels 92, 94, 102,
    105, 106
  hypertension role 105, 106

Vitamin B_6
  deficiency effects
    blood pressure 43–45, 66, 67
    body weight 43, 45
    calcium
      dietary effects 57–60
      uptake by arteries 55–57
    clonidine binding to receptor 50, 51
    convulsions 47
    levels
      γ-aminobutyric acid 42, 45, 50
      dopamine 45, 50
      epinephrine 48
      norepinephrine 45, 48–52
      serotonin 45, 50, 52
      thyrotropin 46
      thyroxine 46
      triiodothyronine 46
    toxemic placenta 42
  seizure role 42, 47
Vitamin D
  calcium homeostasis role 41, 60, 61, 67
  effect
    calcium influx 62–64
    hypertension 64
  metabolism 60, 62
Vitamin E
  antioxidant 41, 65
  deficiency effects 65, 66
  hypertension role 65, 66
  lipid peroxidation protection 65
  membrane integrity role 41